Facts for Family Planning

2012

Table of Contents

Acknowledgments ii

Introduction 1

Chapter 1: Promoting Family Planning 6

Chapter 2: Planning for Families 14

Chapter 3: Delaying First Pregnancy 22

Chapter 4: Spacing Pregnancies 30

Chapter 5: Completing the Family 36

Chapter 6: Understanding Fertility 42

Chapter 7: Family Planning Methods 54

Chapter 8: Family Planning After Miscarriage or Abortion 74

Chapter 9: Unmarried Young People and Unintended Pregnancy 80

Chapter 10: Family Planning and Sexually Transmitted Infections, including HIV 94

Glossary of Terms 107

Selected Resources 111

Acknowledgments

Facts for Family Planning presents a comprehensive collection of key information and messages that anyone can use who communicates to others about family planning. Although a variety of individuals and groups can use *Facts for Family Planning*, it is primarily for those who communicate to men and women who are seeking information about family planning and help in selecting a family planning method. This publication is modeled on the early, popular versions of *Facts for Life*, a book that helped the child survival community communicate consistently about an emerging body of knowledge and best practices.

Facts for Family Planning was developed by FHI 360. Irina Yacobson, Kaaren Christopherson, and Tula Michaelides were the principal writers. Bill Finger was the principal editor, with editorial assistance from Ward Rinehart, independent consultant. Research support was provided by Geeta Nanda.

Victoria Graham from USAID's Office of Population and Reproductive Health within the Global Health Bureau (USAID/GH/PRH) was the lead technical advisor and editor throughout the development of the publication, including the technical content review process.

Jeff Spieler from USAID/GH/PRH served as the lead technical contributor, with other technical contributions on specific issues from these USAID/GH/PRH staff: Gloria Coe, Sarah Harbison, Erin Mielke, Maureen Norton, Lois Schaefer, and James Shelton. Outside of USAID, technical contributors included Victoria Jennings and Jeannette Cachan, Georgetown University's Institute for Reproductive Health; Elaine Murphy, independent consultant; James Foreit, Population Council; and representatives from Jhpiego.

Carly Rounds and Melanie Tingstrom from Design Lab 360 led the design and layout of this publication, with assistance from Brian Campbell and Kay Garcia. Most illustrations were initially developed by the World Health Organization and are used here with permission. The illustrations in Chapter 6 on anatomy were developed by Population Reference Bureau and used with permission. The fistula graphic in Chapter 3 is adapted from the original drawing by Jonathan LaRocca for OperationOF, used with permission.

We wish to thank the following individuals for providing direction for the content of the publication: Iqbal Shah and Suzanne Reier from the World Health Organization, Sadia Chowdhury from the World Bank, and Nuriye Ortayli from the United Nations Population Fund (UNFPA).

We would also like to thank the individuals who reviewed the publication: Amy Tsui, The Bill and Melinda Gates Institute of Population and Reproductive Health, Johns Hopkins Bloomberg School of Public Health; Jane T. Bertrand, Department of Global Health Systems and Development, Tulane School of Public Health and Tropical Medicine; Rhonda Smith, associate vice president of international programs, Population Reference Bureau; and John Stanback, deputy director of research, FHI 360/PROGRESS project.

We would like to thank the following organizations for their contributions to this publication: Population Reference Bureau, Jhpiego, Georgetown University's Institute for Reproductive Health, Population Council, and FHI 360.

Endorsing partners include: Abt Associates; Adventist Development and Relief Agency International; African Medical Research Foundation; Africare; American College of Nurse-Midwives; CORE Group; Curamericas Global; Food for the Hungry; Future Generations; Global Health Action; Helen Keller International; The William and Flora Hewlett Foundation; Interchurch Medical Assistance World Health; International Committee for Research on Women; International Rescue Committee; International Youth Foundation; Jhpiego; John Snow, Incorporated; Johns Hopkins Bloomberg School of Public Health Center for Communication Programs; Marie Stopes International; Population Council; Population Services International; Save the Children; University Research Company, LLC; WellShare International; and World Relief.

©U.S. Agency for International Development (USAID). 2013. *Facts for Family Planning*. Washington, DC: USAID

ISBN: 978-0-9894734-0-8

Suggested Citation: FHI360. 2013. *Facts for Family Planning*. Durham, North Carolina: FHI360/Communication for Change Project

This work was made possible by the generous support of the American people through USAID under the terms of Cooperative Agreement with FHI 360, No. GPO-A-00-07-0004-00. The contents are the responsibility of FHI 360 and do not necessarily reflect the views of USAID or the United States Government.

The Knowledge for Health project, implemented through the Johns Hopkins Bloomberg School of Public Health Center for Communication Programs, is coordinating dissemination of this publication. For more information or questions about *Facts for Family Planning*, please contact:

Knowledge for Health Project– Orders Department
JHU Center for Communication Programs
111 Market Place, Suite 310
Baltimore, MD 21202
Tel: 410-659-6300   Fax: 410-659-6266   Email: orders@jhuccp.org

Introduction

Facts for Family Planning provides key information for those who communicate about voluntary family planning and reproductive health in developing country settings. This book is designed to help in developing materials and messages about family planning.

Program directors and managers can use this information to guide the development of training materials and communication messages for program activities. Counselors, social workers, community health outreach workers, teachers, religious leaders, and others who help individuals and couples make informed decisions about their lives can use this book as a resource for information on family planning. Journalists and media outlets can also use the information here as a basis for television, radio, and other mass media programming and for use in social media applications such as websites or on cell phones.

Facts for Family Planning also offers a resource for those developing targeted advocacy messages and materials for politicians and decision-makers who influence policy and funding for family planning services. It can also serve as a resource for those not familiar with the family planning field when creating communication campaigns designed to promote healthy behaviors.

USING THIS BOOK

Following the format of UNICEF's successful book on child health, *Facts for Life*, each chapter of *Facts for Family Planning* has three parts:

- An **INTRODUCTION** briefly describes what the chapter covers.
- **KEY FACTS TO SHARE** provide main points to communicate to others.
- **SUPPORTING INFORMATION** gives background and details on each of the key facts.

The **key facts** may need to be translated into other languages or adapted to reflect local situations and customs. In doing so, local health experts should review the translation or adaptation to be sure the information remains correct. The key facts can be adapted to many situations and communicated in many ways, for example:

- Designing communication for family planning programs
- Developing family planning counseling materials and tools
- Designing outreach materials and strategies for community groups
- Developing guidance for individuals who talk to family and friends about family planning
- Reporting on family planning for newspapers, radio, and television
- Designing mass media programs that discuss family planning including public service announcements, drama/soap operas, game shows, and social media outlets (e.g., Internet and cell phone applications)
- Advocating policies that support family planning and seeking government commitment for high-quality, voluntary services

The **supporting information** can be especially helpful for developing messages for health workers or anyone else who wants to know more about family planning.

CONTENT OVERVIEW

Facts for Family Planning contains 10 chapters. Chapter 1 presents the importance of family planning to women's health and key reasons why the promotion of family planning is important at the community, national, and international levels. The information in this chapter will be helpful to those advocating for family planning, including journalists. Chapters 2–5 guide couples as they make informed decisions about planning their family, the best time to have the first pregnancy, how to space future pregnancies for the health of the mother, and what steps to take when their family is complete. These chapters will be helpful to those who communicate directly with families or develop communication materials on family planning.

Chapter 6 provides key messages and information that women and men need to know about their fertility. Chapter 7 presents basic information on the most common contraceptive methods.

The last three chapters provide information on important issues related to family planning. Chapter 8 includes key messages about family planning for women who have a miscarriage or an abortion. Chapter 9 focuses on unmarried youth and how messages about contraceptive use and prevention of sexually transmitted infections (STIs), including HIV, can be useful to young people. Chapter 10 provides basic information on family planning as it relates to STIs/HIV.

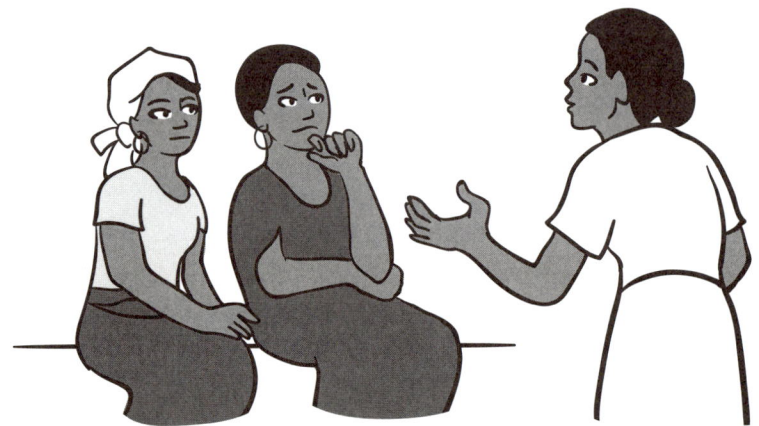

TIPS ON USING THIS BOOK

The key messages in *Facts for Family Planning* need to be adapted so they relate to people's communities, their families, and their lives. This will help people understand, accept, and act on the information presented here. When adapting these messages, users need to take into account a country's customs and traditions. If people feel respected and understand how family planning relates to the health and well-being of their families, they are more likely to follow the advice that *Facts for Family Planning* offers. Please keep the following steps in mind when adapting key messages:

- Identify the people who need the information in *Facts for Family Planning* and the most appropriate practices that need to be communicated. When adapting the message consider the goals, language, customs, and level of knowledge of the people you are working with. Messages that are relevant and easy to understand are more likely to be accepted and acted upon.
- Use common language that people can understand. Create clear messages, and keep instructions easy so they can be followed. Avoid using technical details or words that people will not understand.

- Note that the terms "family planning" and "contraception" are used interchangeably in this book. The term "family planning" works best when talking about couples or when discussing not only the method of contraception but also issues related to family planning information, counseling, commodities, and the health system. However, when discussing issues related to single people and unmarried youth in particular, the term "contraception" or "contraceptive services" is more accurate.
- When developing these messages, try them out first to make sure that the people who receive the information understand it and know how to put the information into action. Gently ask questions about the information and discuss the answers with them to make sure they understand.
- Make the messages relevant to people's lives. Find ways to make the information from *Facts for Family Planning* interesting and meaningful to the specific audience. For example, use local or personal examples to help illustrate the key messages.

Communicating helpful information about family planning will help strengthen individuals, families, communities, and, ultimately, nations. Please share *Facts for Family Planning* with your family, friends, colleagues, and community leaders.

Promoting Family Planning

INTRODUCTION

Voluntary family planning has been widely adopted throughout the world. More than half of all couples in the developing world now use a modern method of contraception for healthy timing, spacing, and limiting of births to achieve their desired family size. Few other public health measures have demonstrated so great a life-saving, health, and economic impact for such a low cost. Family planning has saved the lives of millions of mothers and their children and has improved the well-being of families and communities.

The success of family planning has not been consistent across countries or even within countries. In some countries, the level of contraceptive use has remained low or risen slowly over the years. Even in countries where modern-method use is relatively widespread, there are populations without access to family planning services. In the developing world, an estimated 222 million women would like to space or limit their pregnancies but are not using a contraceptive method. South Asia has the highest number of women who want to avoid pregnancy and are not using a family planning method. Sub-Saharan Africa has the largest proportion of women who fall in this category. The United Nations estimates that the desire to use family

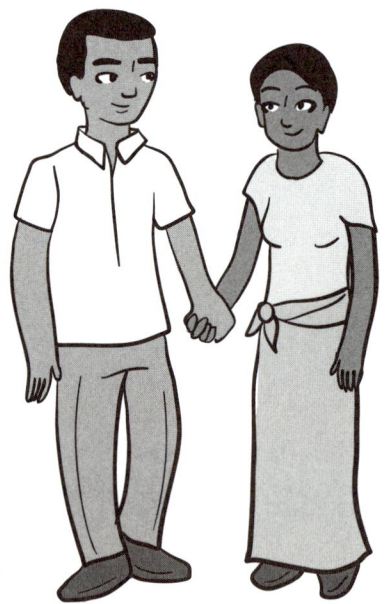

(Continued on page 8)

KEY FACTS TO SHARE: **PROMOTING FAMILY PLANNING**

1. Family planning saves the lives of women, newborns, children, and teenage girls.

2. Family planning lowers the number of unplanned pregnancies and abortions.

3. Family planning benefits families and communities.

4. Family planning benefits nations by enabling increased public spending per person in all sectors.

5. Family planning reduces the burden on natural resources and the environment.

CHAPTER 1: **PROMOTING FAMILY PLANNING**

planning will grow by 40% by 2050, as record numbers of young people enter their childbearing years.

There are some women — and couples — who have access to family planning services and would like to use contraception but do not. These women say that the main reasons for not using contraceptives are side effects, infrequent sex, fear of their partner's disapproval, and religious beliefs that do not support family planning. These concerns can be addressed by trusted persons, such as health workers, religious leaders, friends, and journalists, who communicate key information effectively.

Providing accurate and reassuring information to women and couples about family planning is an essential component of family planning promotion and advocacy. Those who do so do a great service to women, their families, and the community. Effectively promoting family planning will help people to start using contraception and motivate them to continue. This will improve their health and the health of their children. In turn, communities and nations will benefit from stronger, healthier, more productive citizens who can better care for themselves, educate their children, and put less strain on limited resources.

CHAPTER 1: **PROMOTING FAMILY PLANNING**

SUPPORTING INFORMATION

FACT 1.
Family planning saves the lives of women, newborns, children, and teenage girls.

Family planning can significantly reduce the risk of maternal, newborn, infant, and child illness and death by preventing a high-risk pregnancy in women with certain health conditions or characteristics, or by preventing an unplanned pregnancy. Women typically welcome pregnancy and childbirth, especially when planned. However, many pregnancies are unintended or mistimed, and the risk of illness and death associated with these events can be very high.

THE HEALTHIEST TIMES FOR A WOMAN TO BECOME PREGNANT ARE:

- Between the ages of 18 and 34.
- At least 24 months after a live birth.
- At least 6 months after a miscarriage.

Access to family planning information and services prevents unnecessary maternal death or illness due to an unintended pregnancy. There are more than 287,000 maternal deaths a year. For every maternal death, at least 30 other women suffer serious illness or debilitating injuries, such as severe anemia, damage to the reproductive organs or nervous system, chronic pain, infertility, and the inability to control the leakage of urine. If women had only the number of pregnancies that they wanted, maternal mortality would drop by about one-third. In spite of this, about 222 million women in the developing world who want to avoid a pregnancy are not using a modern contraceptive method.

CHAPTER 1: **PROMOTING FAMILY PLANNING**

Health risks associated with childbirth are higher to the mother when she is among those under age 18 or older than age 34. Also, women with five or more children are 1.5 to 3 times more likely to die from complications of pregnancy and childbirth than women with two or three children. Women with more than three children are more likely to suffer from anemia, require blood transfusions during delivery, and die of bleeding than are women with fewer children.

Family planning also saves the lives of newborns and children. About one-third of all infant deaths occur because mothers had births too close together or were too young. Babies born to women under the age of 18 are more likely to be born before reaching full term, to have a low birth weight, and to have problems during birth that could lead to death of the baby or the mother. Family planning helps women delay their first pregnancy until the age of 18 years or older.

After a live birth, family planning helps a woman space her next pregnancy for at least the recommended two years (approximately three years between births). With such spacing, children are more than twice as likely to survive infancy and are healthier. The time between pregnancies also allows the mother to provide the benefits of breastfeeding longer and spend more time with each child. This contributes to the child's physical health and mental and emotional development.

Family planning can also save teenage girls' lives by helping them to delay the first pregnancy. If they become pregnant, girls ages 10 to 14 are five times more likely to die of pregnancy-related causes than women ages 20 to 24. Marriage by girls before the

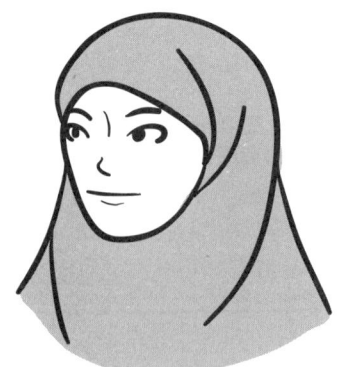

CHAPTER 1: **PROMOTING FAMILY PLANNING**

age of 18 is considered normal in many countries, even though it is against international standards and many national laws. In Ethiopia, for example, half of the girls are married by the age of 18, and one of every four girls is married by the age of 15.

Globally, it is estimated that nearly 10 million adolescent girls marry each year. These young brides are pressured to begin having children even though they are not fully physically developed and their bodies are not prepared for pregnancy. Many young girls marry older men, putting them at higher risk of being infected by their husbands with sexually transmitted infections (STIs), including HIV. Parents and the community should protect these girls by supporting healthy timing of pregnancies and by providing the girls with information and counseling. This support may help them to negotiate, if possible, delaying their first pregnancy until they are at least 18 years old.

Many unmarried girls run the risk of becoming pregnant if they are sexually active. While sexual activity of unmarried girls may not be socially accepted, providing contraception to these young women may save their lives. In addition, delaying pregnancy will allow these young women to complete their education, prepare to join the paid workforce, and contribute to the household income.

FACT 2.
Family planning lowers the number of unplanned pregnancies and abortions.

Each year there are an estimated 80 million unintended pregnancies, and 42 million of these pregnancies end in abortion. The primary reason for abortion is to end an unplanned pregnancy. To reduce the number of unintended pregnancies and thus the number of abortions, women must

CHAPTER 1: **PROMOTING FAMILY PLANNING**

have access to contraceptive information and services. Studies around the world have found that, where women received high-quality contraceptive services, the number of abortions decreased. These studies demonstrate the essential role of contraceptive services in reducing abortions.

FACT 3.
Family planning benefits families and communities.

When couples have only the number of children they want, there are fewer children needing educational and other community services. Healthy children are better able to learn, which puts less strain on teachers and schools. Researchers have shown that personal savings and investments increase when working parents have fewer dependents to support. Family planning results in smaller, healthier families that are better able to care for themselves. The health, education, and public services of communities are less burdened. There are fewer children to immunize and treat. This means health resources can be utilized more efficiently, with less overcrowding in hospitals and at clinics. With fewer children to educate, schools will be less crowded, and teachers will be able to pay more attention to every child. There will be lower demands on clean water, sanitation, transportation, and other public services. By embracing family planning programs, communities strengthen their ability to provide public services and improve the lives of their families.

Family planning is also one of the most cost-effective and powerful strategies to empower women and improve their lives. Women who are empowered to make choices about childbearing are more likely to get better education and job experience, and are more likely to contribute to the economic health of their families and communities.

CHAPTER 1: **PROMOTING FAMILY PLANNING**

FACT 4.
Family planning benefits nations by enabling increased public spending per person in all sectors.

Governments around the world are focused on combating poverty and achieving a range of health and development goals, such as those outlined in the United Nations Millennium Development Goals (MDGs). Family planning contributes to achieving nearly all of these goals. Reducing the number of unplanned births and having smaller families helps to reduce the level of need for public-sector spending in health, water, sanitation, education, and other social services. Preventing unplanned pregnancy among HIV infected women is the most cost-effective way of preventing maternal to child transmission of HIV. Family planning helps nations to reach social and economic goals, beginning at the community level. Family planning is an important and cost-effective investment for governments and contributes to multiple economic and health priorities, including reducing poverty.

FACT 5.
Family planning reduces the burden on natural resources and the environment.

Family planning not only has an impact on the health and well-being of families but also contributes to better management and conservation of natural resources and eases population pressure on local ecosystems. The population level in a country has a profound impact on the demands placed on limited natural resources. Rapidly growing populations increase demand for scarce natural resources and put pressure on water, trees, farmland, wildlife, and ecosystems. Smaller families help to protect natural resources and keep them from being overused and destroyed.

Planning for Families

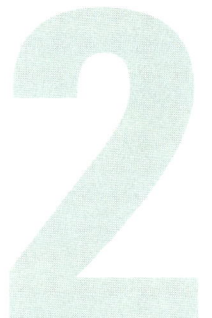

INTRODUCTION

Both women and men have an important role to play in planning a family. However, in some cultures contraception is considered to be a woman's responsibility, so many women make family planning decisions on their own. Ideally, the couple will discuss together how many children to have and when to have them. This communication about having children will help couples think about many issues — such as how they will provide for and raise their children. Health care providers, religious and community leaders, and other who discuss family issues with individuals or couples should help them think through and talk to each other about these important matters.

Couples need to plan ahead and talk about family planning before they start having sex and throughout their relationships as their circumstances change. This requires couples to learn to talk about sex and use contraception if they do not want to get pregnant soon after marriage. Many cultures expect a couple to have children soon after they are married. Counselors need to educate husbands and other family members about healthy timing and spacing of

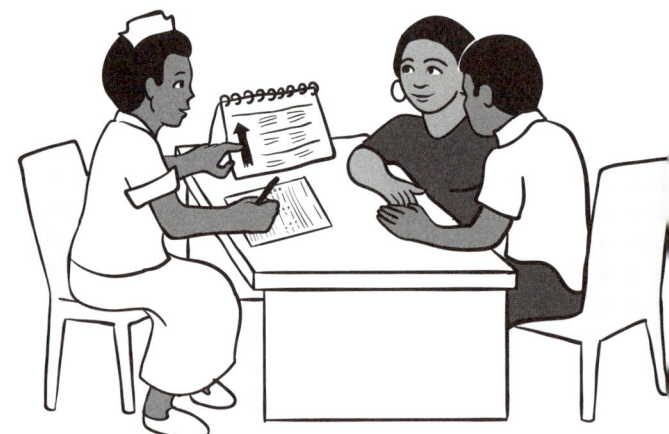

(Continued on page 16)

KEY FACTS TO SHARE: PLANNING FOR FAMILIES

1. For couples, discussing the chance of pregnancy and seeking family planning counseling as soon as possible will help them prevent an unintended pregnancy.

2. Couples will be better able to provide and care for their families if they can decide whether and when to have a child based on their circumstances, including how many children they already have.

3. Family planning enables couples to time pregnancies in a way most beneficial to the mother's and children's health.

4. Men as well as women need to know that contraceptive methods help prevent unintended pregnancies.

5. Those who influence a couple in their decisions about having children need to understand the health benefits of delaying or spacing pregnancies and the importance of having the number of children the couple can provide and care for.

6. Families will be happier and more stable when women and men treat each other with kindness and respect. This respect includes never forcing a partner to have sex and avoiding all forms of violence.

CHAPTER 2: PLANNING FOR FAMILIES

pregnancies and encourage them to support women and couples if they want to postpone pregnancy.

Each pregnancy and childbirth is a good time for a couple to discuss if they have reached a desired family size and what they need to do to space or avoid a future pregnancy.

Young people need to think about the consequences of sex, including whether they are ready to raise a child. Unmarried and married couples may think of pregnancy and family planning in quite different ways. Most of the material in this booklet refers to all sexually active people. Chapter 9 provides information specific to unmarried young people.

Whether or not a couple has discussed family planning, most women visit family planning services alone. Whether women or men come alone or as a couple, they should always be welcomed and served with respect, regardless of age.

WHEN PLANNING A FAMILY, A COUPLE NEEDS TO CONSIDER:

- The healthiest time to have their first child (*see Chapter 3*)
- The healthiest time for the next pregnancy (*see Chapter 4*)
- How many children they can support and when to stop having children (*see Chapter 5*)
- When a woman is most likely to become pregnant (*see Chapter 6*)
- What contraceptive method to use when they need to delay or avoid pregnancy (*see Chapter 7*)

Discussions about planning a family raise issues related to gender roles. Counselors and others talking to couples about having children have an opportunity to promote mutual respect between men and women. Discussing mutual respect involves addressing the difficult issues of violence, including its harmful effects in the home and forcing a partner to have sex against her will.

CHAPTER 2: **PLANNING FOR FAMILIES**

SUPPORTING INFORMATION

FACT 1.
For couples, discussing the chance of pregnancy and seeking family planning counseling as soon as possible will help them prevent an unintended pregnancy.

Typically, when they start having sex, couples do not want to talk about using a contraceptive method. But they need to discuss contraception as soon as possible — and ideally before the start of sexual relations — to avoid an unintended pregnancy. Women and men can visit with a health worker or counselor to learn about contraceptive options and can choose a method that best suits them.

When both partners are involved in the selection of a method, this joint decision will help ensure that they will be happier with the method and will use it consistently and correctly every time they have sex. Ideally, couples will continue to talk together about their ideal family size and seek family planning counseling as life circumstances change.

In many cases a woman seeks family planning counseling on her own or with female friends. She may or may not have discussed family planning with her husband. Some women may worry that their husbands will disapprove, and so they prefer to keep the use of contraception private. A family planning counselor should welcome her and help the woman choose a method that is right for her situation, regardless if she comes with her husband or partner, or by herself.

Men, also, may seek family planning services without their partners. These men should also be welcomed by a family planning counselor and served.

CHAPTER 2: PLANNING FOR FAMILIES

FACT 2.
Couples will be better able to provide and care for their families if they can decide whether and when to have a child based on their circumstances, including how many children they already have.

For the health and well-being of the family, it is ideal for women and men to plan together when and whether to have a child and to take into consideration their life plans, education, desires for their children, and their jobs. This will help a couple make sure they will have enough money to feed, clothe, educate, and provide health care for each of their children.

Below are important questions for a couple to consider when thinking about whether or when to have a child. If a couple can answer yes to all of these questions, they will have confidence that it is a good time — for mother, baby, and family — to try to become pregnant.

- Is the woman at least 18 years old?
- Will the baby be born before the mother is 35 years old?
- Has there been at least two years since the last baby was born?
- Can the family afford to feed and educate another child?
- Does the couple want another child?

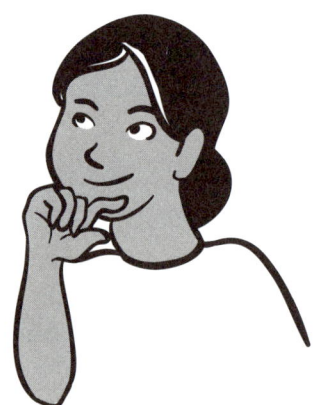

Once a decision has been made to delay or avoid pregnancy, a couple will need information about contraceptive options available to them and where to get family planning services. Those who counsel couples and share information about family planning in the community need to be aware of these important considerations in planning a family.

CHAPTER 2: **PLANNING FOR FAMILIES**

FACT 3.
Family planning enables couples to time pregnancies in a way most beneficial to the mother's and children's health.

Couples should consider the health of the mother and children when planning a pregnancy. Women are in their healthiest years for childbearing between the ages 18 and 34. For the health of the mother and child, a couple needs to plan their first pregnancy when the woman is at least 18 years of age. If a woman is sexually active before age 18, she should use a contraceptive method to protect herself from a potentially dangerous or unintended pregnancy.

Couples should plan for at least two years between the birth of one child and trying to get pregnant again. After a miscarriage or abortion couples should wait six months before the woman tries to become pregnant again. Time between pregnancies allows the woman to regain her strength. This will help ensure that she and her child are healthier and have a better chance to survive.

When a woman is older than 34, the couple should know that pregnancy at this age carries risks for the health of both mother and child. At that age, a woman may want to choose a long-acting contraceptive method or a permanent method — either female sterilization or, for the man, vasectomy.

FACT 4.
Men as well as women need to know that contraceptive methods help prevent unintended pregnancies.

Both men and women care about the health and well-being of the family. Therefore, knowing how family planning can contribute to this well-being is useful to both men and women. When a husband and wife plan how many children they want to have and how to space pregnancies, the man, woman, and children all benefit.

CHAPTER 2: **PLANNING FOR FAMILIES**

Communicating about family planning with men — as individuals, in groups, and as part of a couple — is an important part of promoting family planning. Men need to understand the choices and implications related to contraceptive options. They may choose to support their wives in using a method or consider using condoms or choose a vasectomy. In addition, men of all ages, married and unmarried, have other sexual health needs. They need good-quality services that support them and treat them with respect.

Men, like women, may have concerns about contraception, including how safe a method is, how long it takes for a woman to get pregnant when contraceptive use stops, and how different contraceptive methods may affect the couple's sex life. A family planning counselor can provide men and women with information about contraceptive methods and address specific concerns.

FACT 5.
Those who influence a couple in their decisions about having children need to understand the health benefits of delaying or spacing pregnancies and the importance of having the number of children the couple can provide and care for.

Often, members of the extended family and others may urge a newly married couple to have a child right away or to have children spaced closely together. These individuals, while they may care about the couple, may not be aware of the importance of delaying the first pregnancy and spacing subsequent pregnancies.

Relatives need to know that spacing births sufficiently gives each child a healthy start before the next child arrives and also gives the mother time to recover her strength. Spacing births also helps a couple to be able to provide food, education, and health care for each child — and to nurture each one adequately. The relatives need to understand the value in not pressuring the couple into having children too soon or too close together, and the importance of having the number of children the couple can provide and care for.

CHAPTER 2: **PLANNING FOR FAMILIES**

Communicating this information to relatives and friends is an important element of family planning education. Well-informed relatives and friends can encourage the couple to delay their first pregnancy, space subsequent pregnancies, and have only the number of children for whom they can provide and care for.

FACT 6.
Families will be happier and more stable when women and men treat each other with kindness and respect. This respect includes never forcing a partner to have sex and avoiding all forms of violence.

Both men and women need to understand the harm that results from coercive or forced sex, and violence directed toward women and children. Violence not only causes bodily harm to women but also can lead to depression and even suicide. Violence affects women's ability to care for the family. Children who are victims or witnesses of violence suffer serious emotional damage that can harm their ability throughout their lives to learn and to get along with others.

Women as well as men have the right to consent to sex or to refuse it — without fear of violence. Forced sex, even involving a married couple, may not consider contraception and thus result in an unwanted pregnancy. When men and women treat each other with respect, the family will be happier and more stable.

Attitudes about violence toward women are changing. More and more, men who are most respected in their communities believe that real men do not harm women or children. Communities are becoming less tolerant of violence towards women, including actions by police forces.

Delaying First Pregnancy

3

INTRODUCTION

The age at which a woman has her first pregnancy affects the health and life of a mother and her baby. While pregnancy can present health risks at any age, delaying the first pregnancy until a woman is at least 18 years old improves the chances that the mother and her baby will be healthy.

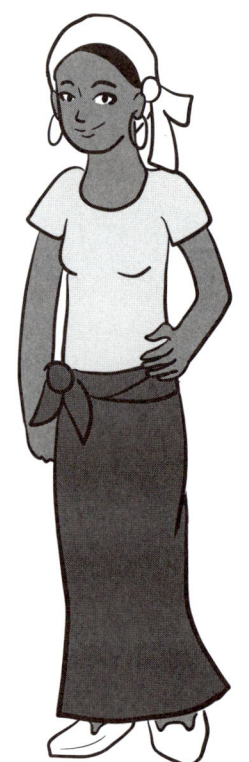

This is important information for young women, their families, and their partners. Counselors can encourage sexually active young women, married or unmarried, to use a contraceptive method to prevent an unplanned pregnancy until they are physically and emotionally ready for childbearing. Counselors should tell young women about their contraceptive options and how to obtain contraceptive methods. They should also talk about STIs/HIV and how to avoid them. This information will help young women and men make good decisions for their health and the health of their future children.

Counselors must welcome single women of all ages who want to use contraceptive services and should not judge them. Regardless of age and marital status, everyone who wants contraceptive information and services should receive them. Withholding services could lead to an unplanned pregnancy, abortion, and even a death that could have been avoided.

(Continued on page 24)

KEY FACTS TO SHARE: DELAYING FIRST PREGNANCY

1. Delaying a first pregnancy until a woman is at least 18 years old is healthiest for both the mother and baby.

2. Because pregnancy poses higher risks of complications for women under age 18, these women need health care during pregnancy. They also need a skilled attendant to oversee childbirth and to care for the mother and child after delivery.

3. Contraceptive methods — other than sterilization — do not permanently affect a woman's ability to have children. These methods can be used to delay the first pregnancy. When a woman is ready to have a child, she can simply stop using the method.

4. Emergency contraceptive pills can prevent pregnancy when taken within 5 days after unprotected sex — that is, when no method was used, a method was used incorrectly, or a method failed.

5. Women's families, including husbands and in-laws, need to be aware that pregnancy and childbirth are often risky for both young mothers and their children. They need to support these young women in postponing pregnancy until they are at least age 18 and their bodies are ready.

CHAPTER 3: DELAYING FIRST PREGNANCY

Young women and men need to understand the social consequences and health risks of teenage pregnancy. Teenage mothers are more likely to be poorer, less educated, have fewer income-producing opportunities, and be more socially isolated than those who delay marriage and pregnancy. To help avoid these outcomes, sexually active young women should be encouraged to use contraception, avoid unplanned pregnancy and early marriage, and stay in school.

Families and other parts of society need to protect girls from unwanted sexual advances that could lead to sexual activity and an early, unwanted pregnancy. Political, religious, and other community leaders can discourage such practices. They can also work with men to help them understand the emotional and physical harm that sexual violence and early pregnancy can cause to young women.

> Withholding family planning services could lead to unplanned pregnancy, abortion, and even death that could have been avoided.

CHAPTER 3: **DELAYING FIRST PREGNANCY**

SUPPORTING INFORMATION

FACT 1.
Delaying a first pregnancy until a woman is at least 18 years old is healthiest for both the mother and baby.

Couples who are sexually active can use a contraceptive method to prevent a pregnancy before the woman reaches the age of 18. Delaying pregnancy until the woman is at least 18 years of age will allow a woman's body to fully mature. Otherwise, she faces a greater risk of complications that can be serious and even fatal.

Complications of pregnancy and childbirth remain a major cause of death in many countries. The youngest mothers face the highest risk. Maternal death rates for young women, ages 15 to 18, are twice as high as for women ages 20 to 24, and girls under age 15 are 5 times more likely to die during childbirth than women ages 20 to 24.

Women under age 18 are more likely to have high blood pressure during pregnancy, which may lead to life-threatening seizures. They are more likely to face other dangers as well, such as severe anemia (low blood iron), bleeding, and infection. Also, because a girl's pelvis has not yet grown large enough for the baby to pass through the birth canal, she often faces prolonged obstructed labor. The pressure resulting from labor that lasts for more than 12 hours can cause the mother a fistula (see box on page 26 for explanation). All these complications may be fatal or cause long-term health problems.

Babies born to women younger than 18 years old are more likely to be born before reaching full term, have low birth weight, and have problems during birth that could be fatal. When they do survive, these children may have life-long health problems.

CHAPTER 3: DELAYING FIRST PREGNANCY

If the couple delays pregnancy until the woman is at least age 18, these complications are much less likely to occur. She will have a much better chance to survive pregnancy and childbirth. Also, her baby will be more likely to survive and to be healthy. In addition, a woman 18 years and older is more likely than a younger woman to be emotionally mature and better prepared to care for her child. In fact, when women wait until age 20 to have their first child, the survival chances and the health of mother and child are even better.

FACT 2.
Because pregnancy poses higher risks of complications for women under age 18, these women need health care during pregnancy. They also need a skilled attendant to oversee childbirth and care for the mother and child after delivery.

All women, but especially women pregnant before age 18, should receive care from a skilled health care provider before, during, and after delivery. Often, health care providers

WHAT IS FISTULA?

Obstetric fistula is an abnormal hole or opening between the vagina and the bladder, or between the vagina and the rectum, or both (see Obstetric Fistula graphic, page 27).

Fistula occurs during childbirth, usually when a woman is in labor too long. Without timely medical intervention or a cesarean section, the baby often dies and the woman is left with a hole that does not heal, causing her to continually leak urine or feces through the vagina. Because of the leaking, she is often abandoned or neglected by her husband and family and ostracized by her community. Without treatment, her prospects for work and family life are greatly diminished.

All pregnant women are at risk of developing a fistula, but especially very young women and women who have given birth multiple times. Three ways to prevent fistula are:

- Family planning to prevent unintended pregnancies
- Skilled attendance at all births
- Emergency obstetric care for those who develop complications

Fistula is also treatable — it can be surgically repaired with a success rate as high as 90% when women have access to a trained surgeon at a hospital providing fistula repair. Fistula is widespread in Africa and Asia.

CHAPTER 3: **DELAYING FIRST PREGNANCY**

OBSTETRIC FISTULA

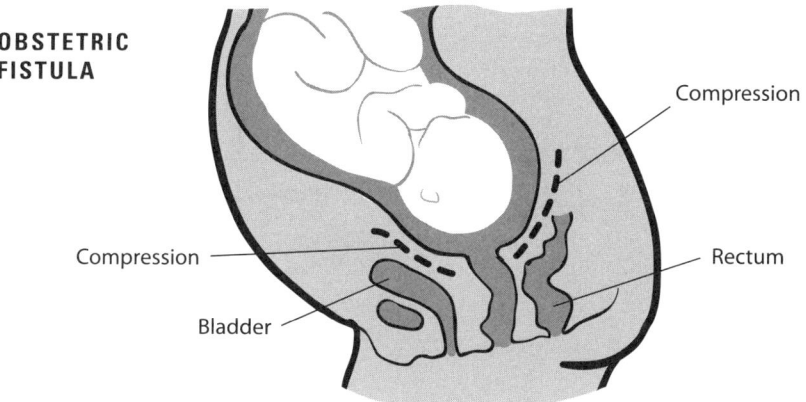

In the graphic above, the head of the baby is shown entering the birth canal. In prolonged labor, the continuous pressure along the compression lines shown above can result in fistula between the vagina and either the bladder or rectum.

can prevent complications. Providers can also either identify and treat or refer for complications and other health problems that may arise for the mother or child. It would be ideal if a young woman would seek health care before pregnancy to make sure her body is fully developed and ready for pregnancy.

Women who deliver before age 18, and particularly those under age 15, are at very high risk for complications during childbirth. To prevent or treat these complications, the young mother and her family should plan to have a skilled attendant on hand for the delivery.

FACT 3.
Contraceptive methods — other than sterilization — do not permanently affect a woman's ability to have children. These methods can be used to delay the first pregnancy. When a woman is ready to have a child, she can simply stop using the method.

Sometimes women and couples do not know what contraceptive methods they can use to postpone or prevent a first pregnancy. Also, they may be

CHAPTER 3: DELAYING FIRST PREGNANCY

concerned that using a family planning method may damage their ability to have children in the future. In fact, women who want to delay their first pregnancy for a year or several years can safely use most family planning methods because they are reversible — "reversible" means that the method does not permanently affect a woman's ability to have children. When a couple decides to stop using the method, the woman may become pregnant soon.

Chapter 7 provides more information on contraceptive methods, including both short-acting and long-acting reversible methods. The chapter also describes the two family planning methods that are not reversible, male and female sterilization. Only couples who want to permanently stop having children should choose sterilization. Couples who want to have children later should choose a reversible method.

FACT 4.
Emergency contraceptive pills can prevent a pregnancy when taken within 5 days after unprotected sex — that is, when no method was used, a method was used incorrectly, or a method failed.

Sometimes women and couples may want to delay their first pregnancy, but are not using any contraceptive method. Some couples use contraception, but may occasionally use it incorrectly, forget to use it at all, or experience method failure (for example, forget to take a pill on time, fail to put a condom on, or the condom breaks or slips). All couples need to know that they may be able to prevent pregnancy even in these cases. Emergency contraceptive pills (ECPs) can help keep a woman from getting pregnant if she uses them within 5 days after unprotected sex. The sooner a woman uses ECPs after unprotected sex, the more effective this method will be. Women should know about emergency contraception and where to get it, so that they can use it quickly if the need arises.

CHAPTER 3: **DELAYING FIRST PREGNANCY**

In some countries health care providers can give ECPs in advance, or a person can buy them at a pharmacy or drug shop. These pills contain the same hormones used in regular oral contraceptive pills. They are very safe, and all women can use them. They are effective only if a pregnancy is not yet established. If a woman is already pregnant, ECPs will not interrupt the pregnancy or cause any harm to the baby. More information on the use of ECPs is in Chapter 7.

FACT 5.
Women's families, including husbands and in-laws, need to be aware that pregnancy and childbirth are often risky for both young mothers and their children. They need to support these young women in postponing pregnancy until they are at least age 18 and their bodies are ready.

The families of a young married woman and her husband need information on the dangers of early pregnancy to the health and survival of the mother and the infant. The families should be encouraged to support the couple's use of family planning at least until the girl reaches the age of 18.

The husbands of many young women are older and may have had previous sexual partners and more chances to get exposed to STIs such as HIV, which leads to AIDS. This raises other issues besides delay of pregnancy, including the possibility of couples being tested for HIV and the need to use condoms in addition to another contraceptive method. More information on using condoms for prevention of STIs/HIV along with another contraceptive method is available in Chapters 7 and 10.

Spacing Pregnancies

INTRODUCTION

Before planning to get pregnant again, couples need to consider the number of children they already have, the impact another child would have on the well-being of their family, and the age of the mother. Couples need to think about how another child would affect the health of all family members, how well the couple can earn and save money, and how each child will be cared for, provided for, and educated. If the couple still wants to have another child, they need to consider the healthiest time for the pregnancy.

It is best for the health and survival of the woman and the child to wait at least 2 years after giving birth before trying to become pregnant again. This message should be shared widely by health care providers, counselors, parents, and other leaders in the community. Using a modern family planning method will make it easier for couples to space their children.

Immediately following childbirth, women can avoid another pregnancy for up to 6 months if they breastfeed only and have not resumed their monthly bleeding. "Breastfeeding only" means giving the baby breast milk and no other liquids or foods, except for vitamins, medicines and vaccines. Feeding a baby

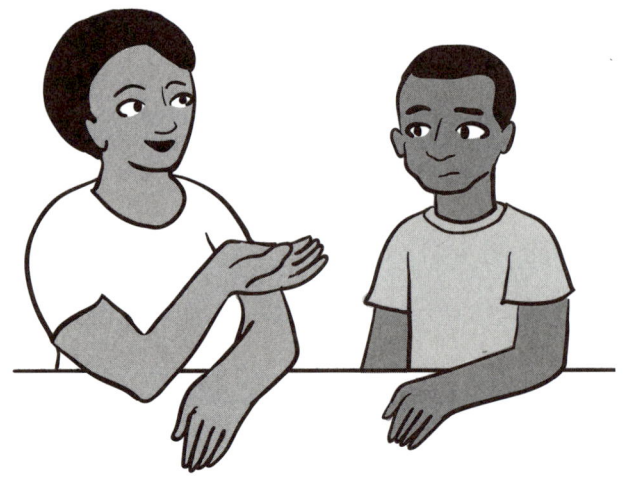

(Continued on page 32)

KEY FACTS TO SHARE: **SPACING PREGNANCIES**

1. A woman should wait 2 years after giving birth before she tries to become pregnant again — by waiting, the mother and her children will be healthier.

2. After delivery, women can achieve protection from pregnancy by breastfeeding only — until their baby reaches 6 months of age OR until their monthly bleeding returns, whichever happens first.

3. If not feeding a baby only breast milk, a woman is at risk of pregnancy as early as 4 weeks after giving birth. To space or prevent the next pregnancy, the couple must start using a modern contraceptive method.

4. During pregnancy a woman and her partner can decide what family planning method to use after the baby is born in order to space or prevent the next pregnancy.

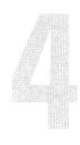

CHAPTER 4: **SPACING PREGNANCIES**

only breast milk provides short-term protection from pregnancy and contributes to infant and child health and survival. Health care providers at all levels should encourage and promote giving a baby only breast milk.

After the pregnancy protection due to breastfeeding ends, women and their partners need to decide on another effective contraceptive method to use. A family planning counselor can provide accurate information about modern family planning methods that can be used after delivery and can help a couple decide what method suits them. Women can choose from many reversible contraceptive methods to delay their next pregnancy. If a woman has had all the children she and her partner/husband want and has completed her family, she or her partner may choose a permanent, non-reversible family planning method. See Chapter 7 for more information on male and female sterilization.

CHAPTER 4: **SPACING PREGNANCIES**

SUPPORTING INFORMATION

FACT 1.
A woman should wait 2 years after giving birth before she tries to become pregnant again — by waiting, the mother and her children will be healthier.

If a couple waits at least 2 years after the birth of a child before trying to become pregnant again, both the woman and her children will be healthier. The mother can breastfeed her older child longer and give the child the ability to grow stronger and better fight disease before a younger brother or sister is born. The next baby will be less likely to be underweight at birth, less likely to become sick as a baby, will have a healthier childhood, and, overall, will be more likely to survive. Waiting for at least 2 years also allows time for the woman to recover from childbirth, regain her strength, and become adequately nourished between pregnancies.

FACT 2.
After delivery, women can achieve protection from pregnancy by breastfeeding only — until their baby reaches 6 months of age OR until their monthly bleeding returns, whichever happens first.

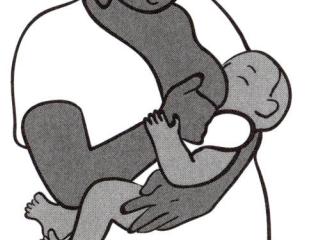

After a woman gives birth, she can avoid another pregnancy for up to 6 months if she has no monthly bleeding and feeds her baby only breast milk. No other foods or liquids should be given, except for vitamins, medicines, and vaccines. The use of breastfeeding only is a short-term family planning method and referred to as the Lactational Amenorrhea Method, or LAM.

CHAPTER 4: SPACING PREGNANCIES

LAM will effectively prevent pregnancy for no more than 6 months. If her monthly bleeding returns, the protection from pregnancy will end sooner, and the women will need another family planning method. Similarly, if the mother starts giving her baby any other liquids or foods and reduces breastfeeding before the baby reaches 6 months old, she must start another family planning method. A couple might want to keep a method such as pills or condoms available at home so they can start it as soon as one of the LAM criteria expires.

Giving the baby only breast milk may be difficult for some mothers in places where it is common practice to give babies other food or liquids at an early age, or where work schedules make exclusive breastfeeding difficult. In these situations women may want to start another family planning method soon after delivery in order to space their pregnancies.

> A woman may be protected from pregnancy if ALL of these three conditions are present at the same time:
>
> 1. The woman breastfeeds only.
> 2. Her monthly bleeding has not returned.
> 3. The baby is less than 6 months old.

FACT 3.
If not feeding a baby only breast milk, a woman is at risk of pregnancy as early as 4 weeks after giving birth. To space or prevent the next pregnancy, the couple must start using a modern contraceptive method.

To space pregnancies for the healthiest outcomes, women who do not feed their baby only breast milk should choose another family planning method and start it no later than 4 weeks after giving birth. These women are at risk of pregnancy as soon as 4 weeks after having a baby, even before their monthly bleeding returns. Most women who are not breastfeeding can start

Facts for Family Planning

CHAPTER 4: **SPACING PREGNANCIES**

any contraceptive method immediately after giving birth. Women who are partially breastfeeding ideally should be guided to choose a method that does not interfere with breastfeeding. See Chapter 7 for information on contraceptive methods.

FACT 4.
During pregnancy a woman and her partner can decide what family planning method to use after the baby is born in order to space or prevent the next pregnancy.

Ideally, a pregnant woman (and her partner) would discuss family planning with a health care provider before she gives birth. This discussion would help the couple be prepared to begin a family planning method at the appropriate time after delivery in order to space the next pregnancy or prevent an unplanned pregnancy.

Pregnancy is a time when many women come in contact with health care providers. This contact offers an opportunity to discuss and choose a family planning method. This counseling before the baby is born is particularly important to give women the opportunity to choose a method that can be provided at delivery, such as immediate post-delivery insertion of an intrauterine device or female sterilization. For such methods, all counseling and decision-making should take place before the start of labor, not on the delivery table.

During a woman's pregnancy is an ideal time for her partner to have a vasectomy, if the couple does not want any more children and chooses that method. Vasectomy takes 3 months to become effective. A man can schedule his vasectomy so that it will be effective by the time his partner delivers a baby and needs protection from pregnancy again.

Completing the Family

INTRODUCTION

Once a couple has reached their desired family size and they do not want another child, their family is complete. Part of this decision is how many children they can provide and care for. It is best for the health of the mother and the child if a couple would have all the children they want by the time the woman reaches the age of 35. Between 18 and 35 are the safest years for childbearing, for both mother and child. Health care providers, as well as community, religious, and political leaders, can educate couples about the safest years for childbearing and how risks for both the mother and the child increase after the woman reaches the age of 35.

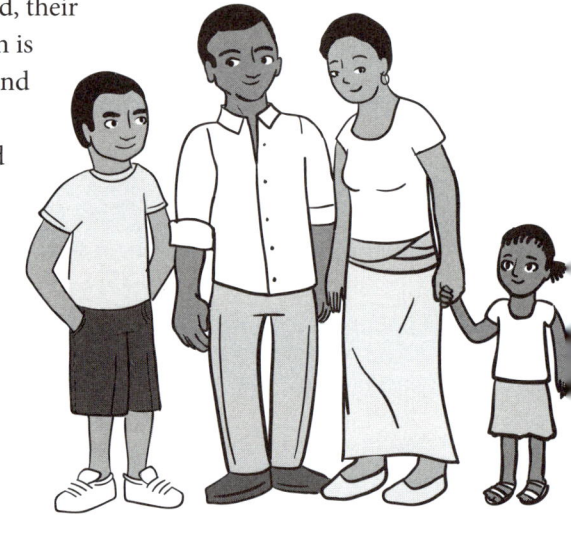

Once a couple has all the children they want, they need an effective contraceptive method that will prevent another pregnancy. Couples can choose from a full-range of contraceptive methods, including a variety of long-acting and permanent methods, as discussed in Chapter 7. But now that the couple has agreed that they have all the children they desire, they may seriously consider and choose a permanent contraceptive method that will provide protection for as long as they are at risk of pregnancy.

KEY FACTS TO SHARE: **COMPLETING THE FAMILY**

1. Having all children before the age of 35 is safer for both the mother and child than having children at a later age.

2. Women and couples who have had all the children they want may choose a long-acting or permanent contraceptive method. These methods are the most effective, and they can provide either many years of protection or life-long protection from pregnancy.

3. Women who are not relying on permanent contraception and want to avoid pregnancy should continue using a contraceptive method until they reach menopause and have not had a monthly bleeding for 12 months in a row.

CHAPTER 5: **COMPLETING THE FAMILY**

SUPPORTING INFORMATION

FACT 1.
Having all children before the age of 35 is safer for both the mother and child than having children at a later age.

The risks associated with childbearing increase as women age and their bodies may be less able to deal with the physical stresses of pregnancy and childbirth. Women over the age of 35 are 5 times more likely to die in pregnancy or childbirth than women ages 20 to 24. They are more likely to have problems during pregnancy such as miscarriage, high blood pressure, and diabetes (high sugar level in the blood). The risk of giving birth to a small baby, a baby with disabilities, or a stillborn baby increases with the age of the mother.

Ideally, a couple should plan to have all the children they want by the time the woman reaches 35 years of age. This may require careful planning because of the importance of spacing births. As discussed in Chapter 4, allowing at least 2 years between giving birth and trying to get pregnant again is best.

Some couples may decide to have a child when the woman is older than 35 regardless of the added health risk. The pregnant mother needs to obtain health care before and after the baby is born. In addition, the baby should be delivered by a skilled health care provider.

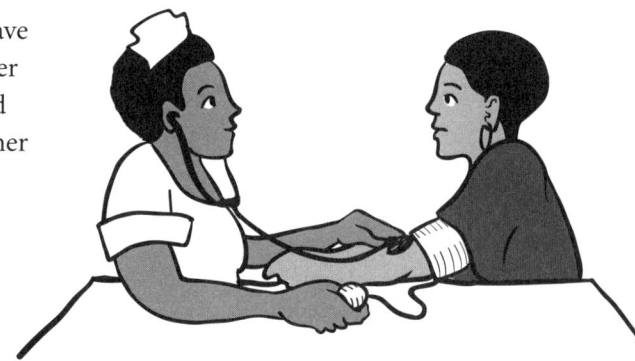

Facts for Family Planning

CHAPTER 5: **COMPLETING THE FAMILY**

FACT 2.
Women and couples who have had all the children they want may choose a long-acting or permanent contraceptive method. These methods are the most effective, and they can provide either many years of protection or life-long protection from pregnancy.

Women and couples who have had all the children they want and consider their family complete can prevent further pregnancies by using the most reliable contraceptive methods. While many methods can be used effectively, the most effective are those that do not require repeated action, each day or each time a person has sex. For example, the copper intrauterine device (IUD) is inserted into a woman's uterus and provides protection for as long as 12 years. Contraceptive implants are inserted under the skin of a woman's arm and provide 3 to 5 years of protection from pregnancy (depending on the type of implant). Once she has an IUD or implant inserted, a woman does not have to do anything more to use the method effectively.

If a couple is certain that they will want no more children, a permanent contraceptive method may be their most convenient option. The permanent methods are female sterilization, also called tubal ligation, and male sterilization, also called vasectomy. Both are relatively simple surgical procedures. Both are very safe and effective. A woman or man who chooses sterilization will be protected from pregnancy for the rest of their lives, although an extremely small risk of pregnancy still exists, if the fallopian tube or vas deferens partially reconnect.

Vasectomy enables the man to take responsibility for preventing unplanned pregnancies. Some men find it difficult, however, to decide to have a vasectomy. Some are needlessly concerned that a vasectomy will reduce their desire for sex or their ability to have sexual relations. And some women are also concerned about how vasectomy may affect their husbands.

CHAPTER 5: COMPLETING THE FAMILY

Counselors can reassure men and their wives that vasectomy does not reduce desire or sexual performance. It may even improve their desire and performance by reducing their worry about causing an unwanted pregnancy. Also, talking with men who have had vasectomies can help a man decide about this method.

FACT 3.
Women who are not relying on permanent contraception and want to avoid pregnancy should continue using a contraceptive method until they reach menopause and have not had a monthly bleeding for 12 months in a row.

As a woman gets older and approaches menopause, her fertility declines. However, a woman should assume that she can still get pregnant until her monthly bleeding stops on its own and she has not had her monthly bleeding for 12 months in a row. Until then, she should continue using a family planning method consistently and correctly. Menopause typically occurs sometime between the ages of 45 and 55.

Continuing to use contraception until menopause involves several important issues. First, as women grow older, they may develop certain health conditions that could make use of some contraceptive methods less safe. A woman who develops a serious new health condition should tell her health care provider what contraceptive method she uses. Her provider should check whether the method is still safe for her and, if not, help her choose another method.

Second, women who have been using a hormonal method — such as progestin-only injectables, implants, or even oral contraceptive pills — may

CHAPTER 5: **COMPLETING THE FAMILY**

have irregular bleedings or a complete absence of bleeding. This is normal with these methods and not at all harmful. However, as a woman approaches menopause, her bleeding patterns naturally become irregular, and bleeding may not come every month. Thus, it may be hard to know whether she already has entered menopause or her absence of periods is due to the hormonal contraceptive.

Therefore, a health care provider may recommend that a woman approaching menopause use a non-hormonal method so that she can monitor her monthly bleeding and know when she has had none for 12 months in a row. Women who choose to switch to a non-hormonal method for this reason must use another highly effective method to prevent an unplanned pregnancy. The copper-bearing IUD is one such method, and it should not be removed until the 12th month after a woman's last monthly bleeding.

Third, aging and menopause do not reduce the risk of STIs. All women, regardless of age, who remain sexually active, should know to continue using male or female condoms if they are at risk of exposure to STIs/HIV.

> When a woman's monthly bleeding has stopped on its own and has not come back for 12 months in a row, it means she has reached menopause. She will not be able to become pregnant again and can stop using contraception.

Understanding Fertility

6

INTRODUCTION

The word "fertile" means the ability to become pregnant or to cause pregnancy. Basic knowledge of both the male and female reproductive systems is important for understanding how pregnancy occurs.

Understanding fertility empowers both women and men to care for their own and others' reproductive health. Everyone needs to know the time during the menstrual cycle when a woman can get pregnant and to know that a man can cause pregnancy at any time.

A woman who wants to become pregnant can use her understanding of her own menstrual cycle to plan sexual relations for the days when she is most likely to become pregnant. A woman who does not wish to become pregnant can avoid sex during her fertile time every month or use condoms during this time each month. Or, she may decide to use a contraceptive method that provides continuous protection from pregnancy for days, months, or years at a time.

Family planning counselors, other health care providers, and anyone who communicates with the public on health issues, need a clear understanding of male and female fertility and should look for opportunities to share this information. Parents, too, can educate their children about fertility and answer

(Continued on page 44)

KEY FACTS TO SHARE: UNDERSTANDING FERTILITY

1. Every month a woman's reproductive system goes through a series of changes called the menstrual cycle. The typical menstrual cycle is about 28 days long; it begins on the first day of her monthly bleeding and ends on the day before the next monthly bleeding begins.

2. In the middle of the menstrual cycle and between monthly bleedings, a woman should assume that there are 12 days when she could become pregnant.

3. Women who are not breastfeeding or only partially breastfeeding can become fertile as early as 4 weeks after delivery and should start using a contraceptive method at that time.

4. Around the time of puberty, a girl's body changes as she develops into a woman. She gains the ability to become pregnant about two weeks before her first monthly bleeding begins.

5. Women in their 40s or older who have no monthly bleeding for 12 months in a row have reached menopause and can assume that they are no longer able to become pregnant.

(Continued on page 45)

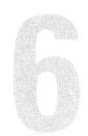

CHAPTER 6: **UNDERSTANDING FERTILITY**

their questions, but they may need support and information themselves. Educators who develop sex education courses or train teachers, and teachers themselves, also need to understand human fertility.

For women, fertility awareness also includes knowing the signs that indicate menopause, the time when a woman's fertility comes to an end and she can no longer become pregnant. This usually occurs between the ages of 45 and 55.

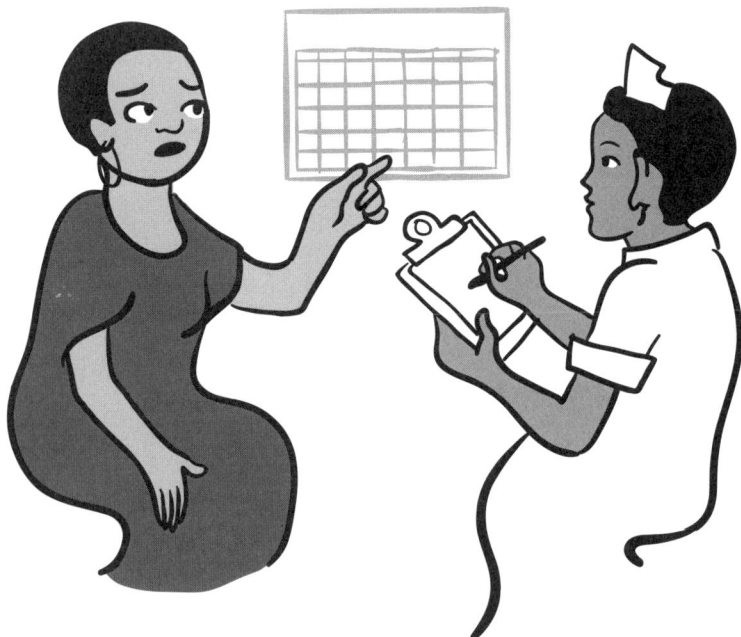

KEY FACTS TO SHARE: **UNDERSTANDING FERTILITY**

6 Around the time of puberty, a boy's body changes as he develops into a man. He becomes fertile and can cause a pregnancy.

7 A man is fertile throughout his life and may be able to cause a pregnancy every time he has unprotected sex with a woman.

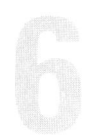

CHAPTER 6: **UNDERSTANDING FERTILITY**

SUPPORTING INFORMATION

FACT 1.
Every month a woman's reproductive system goes through a series of changes called the menstrual cycle. The typical menstrual cycle is about 28 days long; it begins on the first day of her monthly bleeding and ends on the day before the next monthly bleeding begins.

Each month a woman's reproductive system repeats a regular pattern of events that includes vaginal bleeding and is referred to as the menstrual cycle. On day 1 of the menstrual cycle the vaginal bleeding begins — this is also referred to as menstrual bleeding, or monthly bleeding, or a woman's "period." About two weeks later in the menstrual cycle, a woman's ovaries release a mature egg into one of the uterine tubes, also called the fallopian tubes, which lead to the uterus (the womb). At the same time, every month a woman's body builds up a fresh new lining in the uterus. This new uterine lining will nourish a fertilized egg.

If the newly released egg unites with a man's sperm in the fallopian tube — a process called fertilization — the fertilized egg will travel to the uterus and may attach to the uterine lining. There the fertilized egg will grow and develop into a baby. In this case, the uterus will not shed the lining, and the woman will not have her monthly bleeding. If a sexually active woman does not have her monthly bleeding as expected, it is likely that she has become pregnant. However, some women do not have regular cycles, which make it harder for them to know when to expect monthly bleeding. If a woman who is 45 years old or older does not have monthly bleedings it could mean that she has reached menopause and is no longer at risk of pregnancy (see Fact 5 for more information).

If not fertilized, the egg travels to the uterus and dissolves. In this case the fresh new uterine lining is not needed to nourish a baby and is shed. The

CHAPTER 6: **UNDERSTANDING FERTILITY**

uterine lining comes out of the uterus and through the vagina in the form of menstrual blood. This menstrual blood may be bright red, light pink, or brown. It indicates that the woman is not pregnant. A monthly bleeding usually lasts 3 to 5 days. The first day of the monthly bleeding marks the beginning of the woman's next menstrual cycle.

The length of a woman's menstrual cycle typically varies slightly from month to month. Also, the average length of a monthly cycle varies from one woman to the next. Women's cycle length can range from 24 to 37 days, but most women have monthly cycles of between 26 and 32 days, and the average is 28 days.

FACT 2.
In the middle of the menstrual cycle and between monthly bleedings, a woman should assume that there are 12 days when she could become pregnant.

During each menstrual cycle, there are about 6 days in a row when a woman is fertile and can become pregnant. These fertile days are difficult to predict exactly because a woman's menstrual cycles may vary slightly from month to month. However, these fertile days will be immediately before and around the time of ovulation, when an egg is released by an ovary into a fallopian tube.

If a woman has a 28-day menstrual cycle, ovulation will take place mid-way through her cycle — around day 14. Sperm can survive in her reproductive tract for up to 5 days, and the woman's egg can survive not more than 24 hours after ovulation. Thus, she could become pregnant if unprotected sex takes place either 5 days before ovulation or the day of ovulation. This is a 6-day interval that begins around day 9 and ends around day 14 of an average 28-day cycle (see illustration on the following page).

But the length of any woman's monthly cycle may vary from month to month, usually between 26 and 32 days. In addition, ovulation will not

Facts for Family Planning | 47

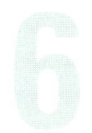

CHAPTER 6: **UNDERSTANDING FERTILITY**

EXAMPLE OF A 28-DAY MENSTRUAL CYCLE: FERTILE DAYS

CALENDAR MONTH							
1 ●	2 ●	3 ●	4 ●	5 ●	6 ●	7	
8	9	10	11	12	13	14 ★	
15	16	17	18	19	20	21	
22	23	24	25	26	27	28	
29	30	31					

● MONTHLY BLEEDING   ★ OVULATION   ▢ INFERTILE DAYS   ▣ FERTILE DAYS

Menstrual cycle length and ovulation time vary from month to month; it is not possible to know the exact days a woman will be fertile. women who want to prevent pregnancy must avoid unprotected sex for a full 12 days — from day 8 through day 19.

occur on the exact same day of every menstrual cycle even if they all are the same length.

Without knowing the exact day of ovulation, it is hard to identify the exact days when pregnancy will be possible. Therefore, a woman should assume there are not 6, but 12 days in the middle of her menstrual cycle when she could become pregnant. These 12 days account for the 6 fertile days that occur in the shortest as well as the longest menstrual cycles. Some women use this information to monitor their cycles and avoid sex or use condoms during the 12 days each month when they may become pregnant as a family planning method.

Several approaches have been developed and tested that use information about the fertile period to avoid pregnancy. These are typically referred to as "fertility awareness" family planning methods, which are described more fully in Chapter 7.

48 | Facts for Family Planning

CHAPTER 6: **UNDERSTANDING FERTILITY**

FACT 3.
Women who are not breastfeeding or only partially breastfeeding can become fertile as early as 4 weeks after delivery and should start using a contraceptive method at that time.

If a woman has had a baby, and is not breastfeeding or is only partially breastfeeding, it may take as little as 6 to 10 weeks for her monthly bleeding to return. However, even though her bleeding has not yet returned, she can be fertile and able to become pregnant as soon as 4 to 6 weeks after childbirth. Just like a girl with her first monthly bleeding, a woman who has given birth may be fertile before her monthly bleeding returns because the egg is released approximately 2 weeks before bleeding begins. The return of fertility following childbirth varies significantly from woman to woman.

> A woman who is not breastfeeding her baby may become fertile as early as 4 to 6 weeks after childbirth.

In contrast, if a woman is breastfeeding, typically she will not have monthly bleedings for several months after childbirth. Women who feed their babies only breast milk until the baby reaches 6 months old will be protected from pregnancy as long as they do not resume their monthly bleeding. If they stop breastfeeding only or if their monthly bleeding returns, they should immediately begin another family planning method to prevent a pregnancy.

FACT 4.
Around the time of puberty, a girl's body changes as she develops into a woman. She gains the ability to become pregnant about two weeks before her first monthly bleeding begins.

Puberty is when the bodies of girls and boys mature into those of adults. Between the ages of about 8 and 13, a girl's body begins to slowly change

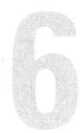

CHAPTER 6: **UNDERSTANDING FERTILITY**

in many ways. Over several years, she becomes taller, her breasts grow and change, and hair grows under her arms and in the genital area. Also, she develops sexual feelings, starts having cervical secretions (wet feeling in the vagina), and her menstrual cycles begin.

A girl's first vaginal bleeding is a clear sign that her menstrual cycles have started and she may now become pregnant. Every month the ovary releases an egg about two weeks before the monthly bleeding begins — *including before her very first period.* This means a girl may be able to get pregnant even before her first monthly bleeding. A sexually active girl going through puberty should use contraception to prevent unplanned pregnancy even if she has not yet had her first period.

Just because a girl has started her periods and she is able to become pregnant does not mean that her body is fully developed and ready to have a baby. In fact, a girl's body usually is not fully ready for pregnancy until she is at least 18 years old. Pregnancy before that age increases the risk of physical complications that can affect the health and well-being of the young mother and her baby. Harmful emotional, economic, and social consequences are also likely to occur if she becomes pregnant or has a baby before 18 years of age.

FEMALE REPRODUCTIVE TRACT

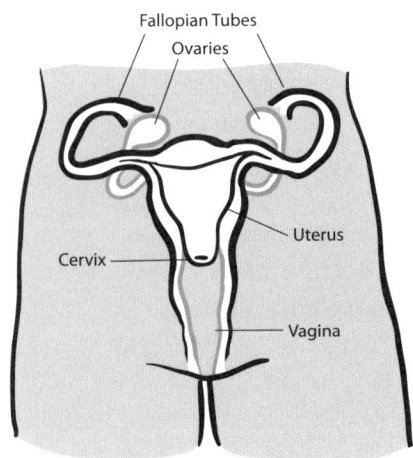

Facts for Family Planning

CHAPTER 6: **UNDERSTANDING FERTILITY**

When a girl is approaching puberty, she must be taught about her menstrual cycle, bleeding, and hygiene. A menstruating girl needs pads, tampons, clean cloths, toilet tissue, and soap and clean water so that bleeding will not interfere with going to school or other daily activities. Support from parents, schools, and the community helps girls get through the time when their bodies are growing and changing and allows them to continue their education. Ideally, by the time a young girl has her first monthly bleeding, she knows what it is and understands that it is normal and a part of growing up.

FACT 5.
Women in their 40s or older who have no monthly bleeding for 12 months in a row have reached menopause and can assume that they are no longer able to become pregnant.

Women's monthly bleeding cycles, which begin during puberty, end at menopause. Menopause happens to most women between the ages of 45 and 55. As a woman nears menopause, she begins to have fewer and less regular monthly bleedings. After a few years she stops having monthly bleeding altogether. When a woman has not had her monthly bleeding for 12 months in a row, she has reached menopause and can assume that she is no longer able to become pregnant.

To avoid an unplanned pregnancy when a woman approaches menopause, a couple should use a contraceptive method until she has had no monthly bleeding for 12 months in a row.

Although a woman cannot get pregnant after menopause, she can still get and pass on an STI, including HIV. Women should be advised to continue to use a male or female condom if they are at risk.

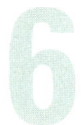

CHAPTER 6: **UNDERSTANDING FERTILITY**

FACT 6.
Around the time of puberty, a boy's body changes as he develops into a man. He becomes fertile and can cause a pregnancy.

When a boy is 9 to 15 years old, his body begins to change. He grows taller and his voice becomes deeper. His penis, scrotum, and testicles become larger. Hair grows on his face, under the arms, and in the genital area. A boy also starts having sexual feelings and sometimes wet dreams, where during sleep his penis gets hard and ejects a thick secretion called semen. This is called ejaculation. The semen contains millions of sperm. Beginning with the first ejaculation, a young man is fertile. Barring certain illnesses and medical conditions, for the rest of his life he will be able to cause pregnancy.

When a man is sexually aroused his penis becomes larger and stiff — this is called an erection. Erection almost always precedes ejaculation. However, men do not need to ejaculate semen each time they have an erection. Not ejaculating semen during an erection does not cause any harm to his body or to his emotional well-being. Ejaculation into a woman's vagina during sexual intercourse may lead to pregnancy.

Although boys become physically able to cause pregnancy, they are not ready to be fathers. Both men and women have a responsibility to care for their children. Bringing a child into the world is a big responsibility, and both parents' maturity is very important.

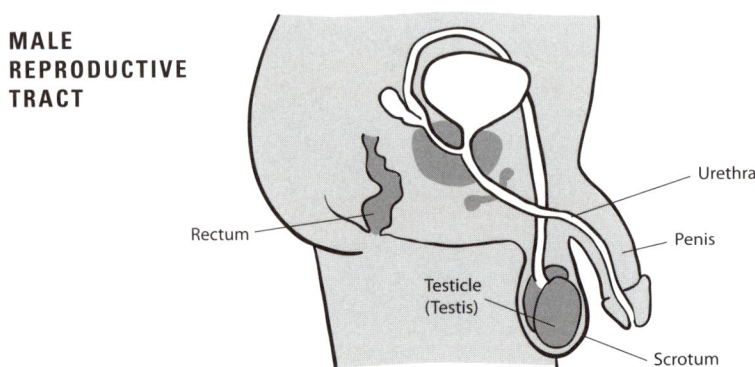

MALE REPRODUCTIVE TRACT

CHAPTER 6: **UNDERSTANDING FERTILITY**

FACT 7.
A man is fertile throughout his life and may be able to cause a pregnancy every time he has unprotected sex with a woman.

MAN'S SPERM DETERMINES SEX OF A BABY

The sex of a baby is determined by two chromosomes that come from the woman's egg and man's sperm. Chromosomes are tiny structures that contain all biological characteristics that are passed to a baby, including the sex of the baby. The chromosomes that determine a baby's sex are called the "X" and "Y" chromosomes. A baby gets one sex chromosome from the mother and one from the father. A woman's egg carries two "X" chromosomes, which are the "girl" chromosomes. The father has one X chromosome and one Y chromosome. If the fertilized egg gets the father's Y chromosome, the baby will be a boy; if the egg gets the father's X chromosome, the baby will be a girl. Thus, the man's sperm, not the woman's egg, determines the baby's sex.

Most men can father a child from the time they have their first ejaculation at puberty and for the rest of their lives, although their fertility may diminish somewhat with age. Also, men are fertile without interruption throughout the month. In contrast, a woman can become pregnant only on certain days of each menstrual cycle.

The man's sperm — not the woman's egg — determines whether the child will be a boy or a girl (see box). Those discussing family planning messages should note this fact because of the potential blame that women face when they do not produce a male offspring. This blaming can lead to dramatic actions such as divorce or violence.

Another message to communicate is that some men are not able to cause pregnancy due to medical conditions that result in very low amount of sperm in the semen. This is important because when a woman does not get pregnant, it is not necessarily her fault. Researchers estimate that infertility in couples may be caused by the man 30% to 50% of the time, depending on the country.

Family Planning Methods

INTRODUCTION

Women, men, or couples can choose from many contraceptive methods to help them plan their family and prevent an unplanned pregnancy. They need to know that if they are having sex regularly and do not use a contraceptive method, about 8 of every 10 women will become pregnant during the next 12 months.

Different people want different things from a contraceptive method. Some want a method that guarantees there is no chance of pregnancy. Some want a quick return to fertility so they can get pregnant soon after stopping a contraceptive method. Some do not want to think about contraceptives every time they have sex. Some do not want to depend on their partner for the success of the method. Some women do not want to remember to take a daily pill, while others find that is easy.

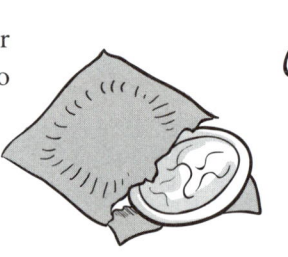

MALE CONDOM   **FEMALE CONDOM**

And there are still other factors that influence method choice. Some may need protection from STIs and will choose condoms to be used alone or in addition to another contraceptive method. Some people want a method

(Continued on page 56)

Only male and female condoms provide good protection against STIs/HIV. No other contraceptive method should be used for this purpose.

54 | Facts for Family Planning

KEY FACTS TO SHARE: **FAMILY PLANNING METHODS**

1. Hormonal contraceptive methods include oral contraceptives pills, injectables, and implants. They all prevent pregnancy mainly by stopping a woman's ovaries from releasing eggs. Hormonal methods contain either one or two female sex hormones that are similar to the hormones naturally produced by a woman's body.

2. Oral contraceptive pills should be taken one pill every day. They are most effective when no pills are missed, the pill is taken at the same time every day, and each new pack of pills is started without a delay.

3. Injectable contraceptives are given by injection into a woman's arm or buttocks once every 1, 2, or 3 months, depending on the type of injectable. Injectables are most effective when women remember to come back for re-injection on time.

4. Contraceptive implants are inserted under the skin of a woman's upper arm and provide continuous, highly effective pregnancy protection for 3 to 5 years, depending on the type of implant. When this time is over, new implants can be inserted during the same visit that the old set is removed.

(Continued on page 57)

CHAPTER 7: FAMILY PLANNING METHODS

they can always get easily whenever they need more. Some people prefer fertility awareness methods because of religious beliefs, because they are worried about side effects, or do not like other methods. Some women want a method that their partner will not know they are using. A few may have a medical condition that could affect the safe use of a particular method.

For many people, the effectiveness of a family planning method is important. The chart below compares the effectiveness of methods as commonly used. The most effective methods are grouped at the top, and less effective methods are at the bottom.

METHOD EFFECTIVENESS ↑

	TYPE OF METHOD			
Best	Implants	IUD	Female Sterilization	Vasectomy
Better	Injectables	LAM	Pills	
Good	Male Condoms	Female Condom	Fertility Awareness Methods	
Least	Withdrawal	Spermicides		

Providers can help women, men, and couples think about their preferences and their situations and choose the method that best suits them. Many women seeking family planning services already know which method they want, and counselors should provide this method along with accurate and complete information, either themselves or through a referral. It is the provider's job to ensure that a client makes an informed voluntary choice and is not denied a method. In rare cases, a client may have a medical condition that will affect which method they can safely use.

KEY FACTS TO SHARE: **FAMILY PLANNING METHODS**

5   Emergency contraceptive pills (ECPs) can help prevent pregnancy if taken within 5 days after unprotected sex. The sooner they are taken, the more effective they are. They are NOT meant to be used for ongoing contraception, in place of a regular method.

6   Intrauterine contraceptive devices (IUDs or IUCDs) are small, flexible plastic devices that are inserted into the woman's uterus. The most common IUDs contain copper, and they work by preventing sperm from reaching an egg. Depending on the type, IUDs can provide protection for 5 to 12 years.

7   Barrier methods are either devices (male and female condoms) that physically block sperm from reaching an egg, or chemicals (spermicides) that kill or damage the sperm in the vagina. The effectiveness of barrier methods greatly depends on people's ability to use them correctly every time they have sex.

8   Fertility awareness methods require a couple to know the fertile days of the woman's menstrual cycle — the days when pregnancy is most likely to occur. During these fertile days the couple must avoid sex or use a barrier method to prevent pregnancy.

(Continued on page 58)

KEY FACTS TO SHARE: **FAMILY PLANNING METHODS**

9 Breastfeeding provides contraceptive protection for the first 6 months after delivery if certain conditions are met. This approach is called the Lactational Amenorrhea Method or LAM.

10 Withdrawal involves a man withdrawing his penis during sex and releasing his ejaculate, which contains sperm, outside the woman's vagina. For most people withdrawal is one of the least effective contraceptive methods.

11 Female and male sterilization are permanent methods of contraception. Sterilization involves a relatively simple surgical procedure that provides life-long protection against pregnancy. Sterilization is appropriate for men and women who are certain they do not want more children.

CHAPTER 7: **FAMILY PLANNING METHODS**

SUPPORTING INFORMATION

FACT 1.
Hormonal contraceptive methods include oral contraceptives pills, injectables, and implants. They all prevent pregnancy mainly by stopping a woman's ovaries from releasing eggs. Hormonal methods contain either one or two female sex hormones that are similar to the hormones naturally produced by a woman's body.

Hormonal methods are highly effective in preventing pregnancies, and nearly all women can use them. All hormonal methods work by preventing the woman's ovaries from releasing an egg every month. Without an egg, there is nothing for sperm to join with — known as fertilizing the egg — so pregnancy cannot occur. They also cause the mucus produced by the cervix to become very thick which prevents sperm from entering the uterus.

Hormonal methods include oral contraceptive pills, injectables, and implants. Each is used differently, has somewhat different side effects, and has slightly different advantages and limitations. It is helpful if a woman talks with a health care provider to make sure she has no health conditions that may make a method unsuitable, to learn the specifics about the method, and to choose one that is right for her. Some hormonal methods are short-acting, and some are long-acting. The short-acting hormonal methods require either taking a pill every day or getting repeat injections as scheduled. They are very effective when used correctly. They are somewhat less effective when women forget to take a pill or to return for an injection on time. Implants are long-acting hormonal methods, and they are highly effective because, once inserted in the woman's arm, the woman will not require further action for 3 to 5 years depending on the implant being used.

> None of the hormonal methods can harm a pregnancy or a baby if accidentally taken by a woman who is already pregnant.

CHAPTER 7: FAMILY PLANNING METHODS

FACT 2.
Oral contraceptive pills should be taken one pill every day. They are most effective when no pills are missed, the pill is taken at the same time every day, and each new pack of pills is started without a delay.

Combined oral contraceptives (COCs). The most commonly used oral contraceptive pills combine two synthetic hormones — estrogen and progestin. These oral contraceptives are often referred to as combined pills or simply "the Pill." If a woman remembers to take the Pill every day, the method is close to 100% effective in preventing pregnancy. However, since some women forget, on average over the course of a year, 8 pregnancies will occur among every 100 women taking the Pill.

Some women experience side effects when first taking the Pill, such as nausea or mild headaches, but the side effects are not dangerous and usually go away after the first few months. Breastfeeding women should delay starting the Pill until the baby is at least 6 months old because the estrogen in the Pill might reduce the amount of breast milk.

Progestin-only pills (POPs). Another type of oral contraceptive pills contains only one synthetic hormone — progestin. These pills are often called progestin-only pills or the "mini-pill."

Progestin-only pills are recommended for breastfeeding women because, unlike estrogen, progestin will not reduce the production of breast milk. Also, progestin-only pills are more effective in breastfeeding than in non-breastfeeding women. For women who are not breastfeeding, the mini-pill may not be as effective as the combined estrogen and progestin pill. The effectiveness depends on taking the mini-pill at about the same time every day.

CHAPTER 7: **FAMILY PLANNING METHODS**

Women who are taking progestin-only pill may experience irregular light bleeding and spotting. This is not harmful, although may be inconvenient for some women.

All oral contraceptives. There is no delay in returning to fertility after a woman stops using either combined pills or progestin-only pills. The Pill is usually readily available at pharmacies as well as clinics, and from community-based providers.

FACT 3.
Injectable contraceptives are given by injection into a woman's arm or buttocks once every 1, 2, or 3 months, depending on the type of injectable. Injectables are most effective when women remember to come back for re-injection on time.

Injectable contraceptives are given by injection into a woman's arm or buttocks in either the muscle or under the skin in the fatty tissue, depending on type of injectable. After the injection, the hormone is released slowly from the injection site into the bloodstream. Different injectables require a woman to return for a repeat injection once every 1, 2, or 3 months.

When women always remember to come for re-injection on time, injectable contraceptives are close to 100% effective. However, some women occasionally are late for re-injection. On average, over the course of a year, 3 pregnancies will occur among every 100 women using injectables.

The most common side effects of injectables are bleeding changes. At first, injectables may cause irregular, heavy, or prolonged bleeding, but after

Facts for Family Planning

CHAPTER 7: **FAMILY PLANNING METHODS**

several injections many women stop having monthly bleeding altogether. This is especially common with the 2- and 3-month injectables. Having no bleeding pleases many women, but some may worry that something is wrong or that they are pregnant. They should know that having no bleedings is harmless and does not cause permanent damage to a woman's fertility. It can even be good for some women's health because the absence of monthly bleedings reduces the risk of anemia (low iron level in the blood). Women need to be aware of these side effects in advance so they know what to expect and do not worry.

Depending on the type of injectable, the return to fertility after a woman's last injection is often delayed and may take from 4 to 10 months. A family planning counselor can help a couple to consider return to fertility when they are selecting a method for timing or spacing pregnancies. A woman can get an injection at a clinic or health outpost. In many countries, community-based health workers and pharmacists are able to administer injections.

FACT 4.
Contraceptive implants are inserted under the skin of a woman's upper arm and provide continuous, highly effective pregnancy protection for 3 to 5 years, depending on the type of implant. When this time is over, new implants can be inserted during the same visit that the old set is removed.

Implants are small plastic rods, each about the size of a matchstick. These rods are placed just under the skin on the inside of a woman's upper arm. Implants are almost 100% effective and can provide 3 to 5 years of protection from pregnancy, depending on the type of implant. Women have found implants to be among the easiest family planning methods to use. After implants are inserted, there are no further actions to take or additional costs until they are removed.

CHAPTER 7: **FAMILY PLANNING METHODS**

A woman must visit a trained health care provider to have implants put in her arm or to have them removed. To continue being highly effective, they should be removed and replaced promptly, in 3 to 5 years, depending on the type of implant. A woman will become fertile again and able to get pregnant almost immediately after the implants are removed. If a woman desires to continue to use implants, a new set can be inserted and the old ones do not have to be removed.

Side effects of implants include irregular vaginal bleeding and spotting. Some women's monthly bleedings stop altogether. This pleases many women, but some may worry that something is wrong or that they are pregnant. It is important to counsel women in advance that they may stop menstruating and that this is harmless.

FACT 5.
Emergency contraceptive pills (ECPs) can help prevent pregnancy if taken within 5 days after unprotected sex. The sooner they are taken, the more effective they are. They are NOT meant to be used for ongoing contraception, in place of a regular method.

Emergency contraceptive pills (ECPs) are sometimes referred to as the "morning-after pill" because they are taken after unprotected sex has taken place. They contain either progestin alone or progestin and an estrogen together, like oral contraceptives. However, the hormone dose in ECPs is higher, and a woman takes only one or two pills.

Emergency contraception works like any other hormonal method by preventing ovulation. There is no evidence that ECPs prevent a fertilized egg from attaching to the uterine lining.

CHAPTER 7: FAMILY PLANNING METHODS

ECPs should not be used in place of regular contraception because they are not as effective as most regular methods. They are 75% to 95% effective in preventing pregnancy depending on the type of ECP and on how soon after unprotected sex the pills are taken. Providers should help women who use ECPs to choose a regular contraceptive method for ongoing protection against pregnancy.

> ECPs do not protect against pregnancy resulting from sex that happens after ECPs have been taken.

ECPs have no serious side effects. Some women may have headaches, nausea, or vomiting after taking ECPs, but these go away within several days. The ECPs that contain only progestin cause fewer side effects and are more effective. There is no delay in return to fertility after taking ECPs. Because of this, ECPs prevent pregnancy only after unprotected sex that occurred within the previous 5 days. ECPs will not prevent pregnancy resulting from unprotected sex that takes place after ECPs have been taken.

ECPs offer women a second chance to prevent pregnancy after unprotected sex. They do not cause an abortion, and, if taken accidentally by a woman who is already pregnant, they will not harm the woman or the fetus or disrupt the course of pregnancy.

FACT 6.
Intrauterine contraceptive devices (IUDs or IUCDs) are small, flexible plastic devices that are inserted into the woman's uterus. The most common IUDs contain copper, and they work by preventing sperm from reaching an egg. Depending on the type, IUDs can provide protection for 5 to 12 years.

CHAPTER 7: **FAMILY PLANNING METHODS**

An IUD is a small, often T-shaped plastic device that is wrapped in copper or contains a progestin hormone. A specially trained health care provider inserts the IUD into the uterus. A plastic string tied to the end of the IUD hangs down through the cervix into the vagina. A woman can check that the IUD is in place by feeling for this string inside the vagina. A health care provider uses the string to remove the IUD when the woman wants it removed or it eventually needs to be replaced. Women who are not pregnant can have an IUD inserted any time. After childbirth, women can have an IUD inserted immediately or within the first two days. If not, she will need to wait four to six weeks to do so.

IUDs are nearly 100% effective. They are long-acting, too. Once in place, they can provide 5 to 12 years of protection from pregnancy, depending on the type of IUD. However, a woman can ask to have the IUD taken out at any time. When the IUD is removed, a woman can get pregnant immediately. Women have found the IUD to be among the easiest family planning methods to use: after it is inserted into the uterus there are no further actions a woman must take and no additional costs until the IUD is removed. Women of all ages can use IUDs, whether or not they have had children. It does not cause infertility.

Women living with HIV can safely use IUDs. However, women at very high risk of STIs or who currently have an active STI, such as gonorrhea or chlamydia, should not have an IUD inserted. The process of inserting the IUD could push gonorrhea and chlamydia higher into the reproductive tract causing a more serious health problem. These infections should be treated and cured prior to IUD insertion.

Copper-bearing IUD. The copper-bearing IUD works by creating an environment in the uterus that damages the sperm and keeps them from uniting with an egg. It is effective for up to 12 years. The most common side effects of the copper IUD include heavier and longer monthly bleeding,

Facts for Family Planning

CHAPTER 7: **FAMILY PLANNING METHODS**

which may be accompanied by increased cramping. For most women these side effects diminish or disappear after the first 3 to 6 months of IUD use.

Hormonal IUD. A hormonal IUD very slowly and continuously releases a small amount of a progestin hormone. It works by thickening the cervical mucus, making it hard for sperm to pass from the vagina into the uterus. It also prevents ovulation in some women and keeps the lining of the uterus from growing.

Once in place in the woman's uterus, the hormonal IUD is highly effective and can be used for up to 5 years. The hormonal IUD also changes bleeding patterns, in this case a woman bleeds less and on fewer days, and the bleeding could be irregular. In fact, many women have no bleeding at all after several months of using this method. Lighter bleeding is a benefit to many women, particularly those with anemia.

FACT 7.
Barrier methods are either devices (male and female condoms) that physically block sperm from reaching an egg, or chemicals (spermicides) that kill or damage the sperm in the vagina. The effectiveness of barrier methods greatly depends on people's ability to use them correctly every time they have sex.

The most common barrier family planning method is the male condom. *Male and female condoms are the only contraceptive methods that provide protection from STIs, including HIV, in addition to pregnancy.* Less common barrier methods are diaphragms and cervical caps; they are not readily available in many countries. All of these devices form a mechanical barrier between the sperm and an egg. Finally, spermicides are chemical substances placed in the vagina — a foam, a gel, film, or a tablet, for example. Spermicides work by killing or disabling sperm.

CHAPTER 7: **FAMILY PLANNING METHODS**

Barrier methods should be used every time a couple has sex. The effectiveness of barrier methods depends greatly on people's ability to use them consistently and correctly. If a woman is fertile and does not use the method consistently and correctly, she can become pregnant.

Male condom. A male condom is a covering — usually made of thin latex rubber — that unrolls over a man's erect penis. It prevents a man's sperm from entering the woman's vagina. It also can keep the small organisms that cause some STIs/HIV from infecting the partner. When condoms are used correctly at every sexual act, they are 98% effective in preventing pregnancy. However, as commonly used, when men sometimes forget or refuse to put a condom on, condoms are only 85% effective. This means that each year out of 100 women who rely on condoms, 15 may become pregnant. Condoms have no general side effects, but a small percent of people may be allergic to latex. These people can use plastic condoms, which are becoming more available in many countries.

Condoms are the only family planning method that provides protection from STIs, including HIV, in addition to pregnancy.

Female condom. A female condom is a lubricated pouch made of thin, soft plastic that fits loosely inside a woman's vagina. It prevents pregnancy by keeping sperm out of the vagina. In addition to preventing pregnancy, female condoms also block transmission of some STIs/HIV. Female condoms are about as effective as the male condom if used consistently and correctly every time she has sex, but less effective as commonly used.

Some women need to practice using the female condom correctly. A family planning counselor can provide clear instructions on how to insert a female condom into the vagina. While a woman can make a decision to use a

CHAPTER 7: FAMILY PLANNING METHODS

female condom herself, it is better if the man also agrees so that they will use it correctly every time. Studies have found that most men do not object to using the female condom to protect against pregnancy and to block transmission of STIs/HIV.

Spermicides. Spermicides are chemical substances that are inserted deep into the vagina shortly before sex to kill or disable sperm. They can be used alone as well as with diaphragms, cervical caps, and condoms. Spermicides are available as foaming tablets, vaginal suppositories, foam, melting film, jelly, and cream.

Used alone, spermicides are one of the least effective contraceptive methods. Even when used consistently and correctly, their effectiveness is only about 82%. Thus, 18 in every 100 women who use spermicides may become pregnant over a year. As commonly used, 29 of every 100 spermicide users will become pregnant within one year of use. Women and couples who want reliable protection from pregnancy should consider other contraceptive methods. Spermicides provide no protection from STIs/HIV and may even increase the risk of HIV if used several times a day.

FACT 8.
Fertility awareness methods require a couple to know the fertile days of the woman's menstrual cycle – the days when pregnancy is most likely to occur. During these fertile days the couple must avoid sex or use a barrier method to prevent pregnancy.

Fertility awareness methods are based on understanding the female and the male reproductive systems. These methods require that couples identify the days when the woman is fertile and may become pregnant and consistently abstain from unprotected sex on those days. Couples who use these methods say they like them because they have no side effects and they do not require procedures, devices, or hormones.

Facts for Family Planning

CHAPTER 7: **FAMILY PLANNING METHODS**

There are two types of fertility awareness methods that help determine fertile days. One uses the calendar to track fertile days, and the other observes the physical signs of fertility. The Standard Days Method (SDM) is the most common calendar-based method and is described below.

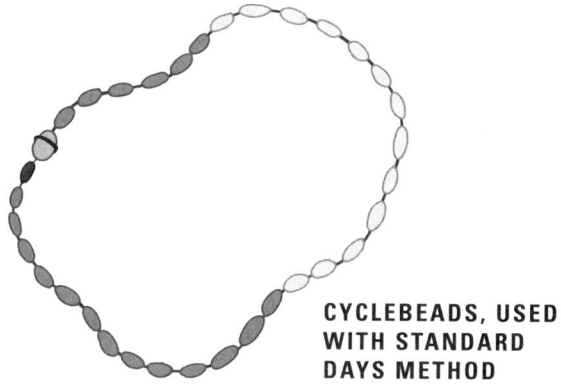

CYCLEBEADS, USED WITH STANDARD DAYS METHOD

To successfully use fertility awareness methods to prevent pregnancy requires a partner's cooperation; men should be willing to abstain from sex or to use condoms on fertile days. Thus, for these methods to be effective, men must become full partners in the decision to use them.

Standard Days Method. To use SDM, the couple avoids unprotected sex from day 8 through day 19 of every cycle, counting the first day of monthly bleeding as day 1. These are the days when the woman is most likely to become pregnant. During that time couples can choose either to abstain from sex or to use a condom or another barrier method to prevent pregnancy.

Many women or couples use CycleBeads (see graphic above) to keep track of their fertile days. CycleBeads are a string of beads that are color-coded to represent different days of the menstrual cycle. The different colors show the days the woman is likely to be fertile and get pregnant and the days when it is safe to have unprotected sex. Others use a calendar to mark those days. Many couples report that they communicate better with each other as a result of using this method. A woman can use SDM if most of her menstrual cycles are 26 to 32 days long. If she has more than two longer or shorter cycles in a year, SDM will be less effective for her and she should consider another fertility awareness method or other modern method.

CHAPTER 7: **FAMILY PLANNING METHODS**

FACT 9.
Breastfeeding provides contraceptive protection for the first 6 months after delivery if certain conditions are met. This approach is called the Lactational Amenorrhea Method or LAM.

The natural effect of feeding only breast milk to a baby delays the return of fertility up to 6 months. For the LAM method to be effective at preventing pregnancy, three conditions must apply:

1. A woman must feed her baby only breast milk

2. The baby is younger than 6 months

3. The mother's monthly bleeding does not resume.

For LAM, feeding the baby "only breast milk" means not giving any other liquids or foods, except for vitamins, medicines, and vaccines. Also, the woman needs to be breastfeeding the baby on demand day and night. If she starts giving any other foods before her baby is 6 months old or if her monthly bleeding resumes, the woman should immediately begin another family planning method to prevent a pregnancy. LAM is 98% effective when practiced correctly.

> A mother should start a family planning method no later than 4 weeks after giving birth to prevent a pregnancy if she is feeding her baby anything other than breast milk.

In addition to protecting against pregnancy, breastfeeding benefits mothers by helping the uterus to contract and return to its pre-pregnancy state, and by strengthening mother-baby bonding. Also, feeding babies only breast milk for the first 6 months of life provides them with the most nutritious food and many health benefits. Since breastfeeding is so important for the health and

CHAPTER 7: **FAMILY PLANNING METHODS**

nutrition of the baby, the mother should consider continuing to breastfeed even when she starts using another family planning method.

The return to fertility after childbirth varies among women and is difficult to predict. A woman who does not breastfeed her baby or breastfeeds only occasionally should assume that she may become fertile as early as 4 weeks after giving birth. To prevent a risky and unplanned pregnancy, she should start a family planning method 4 weeks after giving birth.

FACT 10.
Withdrawal involves a man withdrawing his penis during sex and releasing his ejaculate, which contains sperm, outside the woman's vagina. For most people withdrawal is one of the least effective contraceptive methods.

A man uses withdrawal when he pulls his penis out of his partner's vagina while having sex and ejaculates outside the vagina, so that no sperm can enter her body. Withdrawal is less effective than most other methods. As commonly used, it is only 73 percent effective, meaning that 27 of every 100 women whose partners use withdrawal will become pregnant over a year.

Effective practice of withdrawal requires men to have good self-control. A man must be able and willing to withdraw the penis and ejaculate outside the woman's body. If he does not withdraw before ejaculating, his partner may become pregnant. Also, a small amount of semen may be released into the vagina before the full ejaculation, possibly without the man realizing it. Even this small amount of semen may contain enough sperm to possibly cause a pregnancy and to transmit STIs/HIV.

CHAPTER 7: **FAMILY PLANNING METHODS**

FACT 11.
Female and male sterilization are permanent methods of contraception. Sterilization involves a relatively simple surgical procedure that provides life-long protection against pregnancy. Sterilization is appropriate for men and women who are certain they do not want more children.

The permanent methods of contraception are female sterilization, also called tubal ligation, and male sterilization, also called vasectomy. Both methods involve minor surgery. This surgery is very safe and in most cases does not require hospitalization.

Female and male sterilization are close to 100% effective and are considered permanent methods of contraception, although a small risk of pregnancy still remains. Once a woman or man has the procedure, it is very likely that she or he cannot have any more children because generally the procedure cannot be reversed. The couple must talk over the decision to use a permanent method carefully and be certain that they will not want more children. Men and women should understand that other highly effective and reversible contraceptive methods are available if they are not ready for a permanent method. They should discuss the decision with a family planning provider, who will make sure that their decision is voluntary, conduct a physical examination, and decide with the client on a good time to have the sterilization done. A provider can also reassure men and women that sterilization does not affect sexual function and does not make men less masculine or women less feminine.

Female sterilization. Female sterilization is a relatively simple surgical procedure. A very small incision is made in a woman's abdomen, and her fallopian tubes are cut and blocked so that eggs cannot move through the tubes to meet the sperm. Female sterilization has no side effects, and complications are extremely rare when the procedure is performed by a well-trained health care provider. It can be provided almost anytime, including

CHAPTER 7: **FAMILY PLANNING METHODS**

immediately after childbirth, so long as she makes the decision before giving birth. Following surgery, a woman may have some abdominal pain and swelling, which goes away in a few days. If possible, she should return to the health care provider after about a week to have the incision checked for infection and to have the stitches removed.

Male sterilization. Male sterilization — or vasectomy — is an even simpler surgical procedure. A tiny hole is made in the scrotum (the sac that holds the testicles), and both tubes (vas deferens) that carry a man's sperm to his penis are cut and blocked. This keeps sperm out of the semen, the fluid that is released by a man during an ejaculation. The man can still ejaculate and have an orgasm as before, but there will be no sperm in the semen, and so he will not be able to cause pregnancy. Vasectomy has no side effects, and complications of the surgery are uncommon. After the procedure a man may have discomfort, swelling, and bruising in the scrotum. These symptoms usually go away within 2 to 3 days.

Although a man can have sex 2 to 3 days after the procedure, vasectomy is not effective immediately. It takes about 3 months for semen to be completely clear of sperm. During these 3 months a man or his partner should use another family planning method, such as condoms. Or if a woman was already using a family planning method prior to her partner's vasectomy, she can continue using this method for 3 months before discontinuing it. After 3 months a vasectomy is considered effective. Where possible, a health care provider can examine a semen sample under a microscope to see if it contains living sperm. After 3 months, however, this test is not necessary.

Millions of men who do not want more children have chosen vasectomy. Vasectomy is simpler than female sterilization, recovery is quicker — usually a day or two — and the method allows men to take responsibility for family planning. After this procedure, a man can enjoy sex with his partner as before, except now without fear of pregnancy.

Facts for Family Planning

Family Planning After Miscarriage or Abortion

INTRODUCTION

Unintended pregnancy is one of the main reasons that women seek induced abortions. Many unintended pregnancies occur because women cannot obtain family planning information or services when needed. Making family planning information and services widely available to all women and men is the best way to help reduce the number of abortions.

Abortion is the ending of a pregnancy before childbirth. An induced abortion involves intentional removal of the contents of the uterus before the embryo or fetus is able to survive outside of the womb. An abortion can also happen on its own, which is usually called a miscarriage, or a spontaneous abortion. Most miscarriages occur within the first 3 months of a pregnancy.

Women who have had an induced abortion are frequently at higher risk of another pregnancy, which also may be unintended. To help prevent this pattern, health services need to make

(Continued on page 76)

Approximately 1 in 4 women having an unsafe abortion is likely to face severe complications and will seek hospital care, putting heavy demand on scarce resources. For every identified hospital case, there are many other women who have had an unsafe abortion but who do not seek medical care because they fear abuse, ill-treatment, or legal punishment. The World Health Organization estimates that unsafe abortion accounts for 13% of maternal deaths worldwide.

KEY FACTS TO SHARE:
FAMILY PLANNING AFTER MISCARRIAGE OR ABORTION

1 If a woman has heavy vaginal bleeding, fever, abdominal pain, or unusual vaginal discharge after an abortion or miscarriage, she must urgently seek medical care. This may save her life.

2 After an abortion or miscarriage, fertility returns very quickly. To avoid pregnancy, a woman needs to start a family planning method within one week.

3 A woman who wants to become pregnant again after an abortion or miscarriage should wait 6 months so she can regain strength for her next pregnancy.

4 To reduce the risk of infection after an abortion or miscarriage, a woman should avoid having sex until all bleeding stops — usually 5 to 7 days. Women who are treated for infection or abortion-related injury need to be sure the vagina or uterus has healed before having sex again.

CHAPTER 8: **FAMILY PLANNING AFTER MISCARRIAGE OR ABORTION**

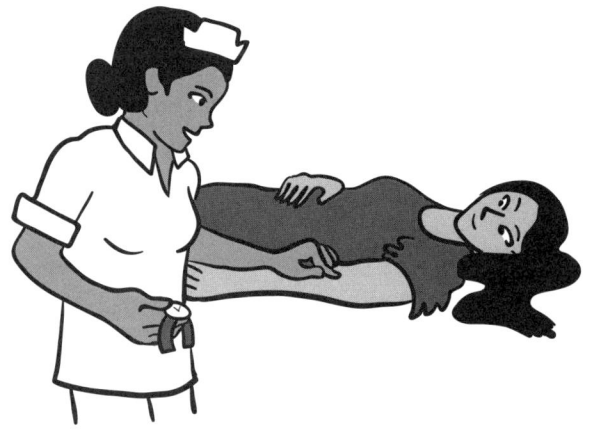

a wide range of contraceptive methods available to women immediately after or when they receive health care for induced abortion or miscarriage.

In some countries women have access to abortion legally, while in other countries abortion is illegal. In both settings, some women obtain abortions from unskilled persons or try to abort themselves. These abortions are unsafe and often dangerous. They may cause infertility and severe and sometimes permanent health problems or even death. Women need to be aware of how dangerous an unsafe abortion can be, and encouraged to use contraception to avoid such a situation. Both women and health care providers need to know the signs of the complications of abortion and miscarriage and the importance of immediate medical care. During post-abortion care, health care providers should offer contraception to women. Family planning should be an essential part of post-abortion care.

CHAPTER 8: **FAMILY PLANNING AFTER MISCARRIAGE OR ABORTION**

SUPPORTING INFORMATION

FACT 1.
If a woman has heavy vaginal bleeding, fever, abdominal pain, or unusual vaginal discharge after an abortion or miscarriage, she must urgently seek medical care. This may save her life.

After an abortion or miscarriage, a woman should seek medical care immediately if she has:

- Vaginal bleeding that is much heavier than the woman's normal monthly bleeding
- Fever or chills
- Dizziness or fainting
- Severe stomach or abdominal pain
- Bad-smelling discharge from the vagina.

If not promptly treated, complications of abortion or miscarriage can cause serious ongoing health problems and leave a woman unable to have children in the future. An abortion or miscarriage can even cause death. Symptoms of these complications include: vaginal bleeding that is much heavier than the woman's normal monthly bleeding, fever or chills, dizziness or fainting, severe stomach or abdominal pains, and bad-smelling discharge from the vagina. A woman who has any of these symptoms after an abortion or miscarriage should seek medical care at once from a trained health care provider.

There are, however, many reasons that women with these complications do not seek immediate medical care, such as the following:

- The woman does not realize that there is a problem. For example, she may think that heavy bleeding is normal after an abortion or miscarriage.
- She does not have the power or ability to seek care, she does not have the money to pay for care, or she has no transportation.
- She hesitates to seek care because she received poor or unfriendly care in the past.
- She does not want anyone to know that she had an abortion or miscarriage.

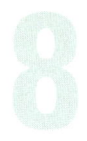

CHAPTER 8: **FAMILY PLANNING AFTER MISCARRIAGE OR ABORTION**

Thus, educating family members and the community about these signs is important. It may be the woman's mother, sister, husband, or friend who first realizes that the woman needs immediate medical care.

FACT 2.
After an abortion or miscarriage, fertility returns very quickly. To avoid pregnancy, a woman needs to start a family planning method within one week.

A woman's ability to become pregnant returns as early as 2 weeks after an abortion or miscarriage — before her monthly bleeding begins. To prevent another pregnancy, she needs to start a family planning method immediately or at least no later than one week after an abortion. Even if her pregnancy was planned and she wants to get pregnant again, she needs to begin using a contraceptive method to give her body time to regain its strength and prepare for the next pregnancy. Ideally, the woman should receive counseling and a contraceptive method before she leaves the clinic.

> Health care providers can help a woman to avoid future abortions by helping her understand why the unintended pregnancy occurred and helping her select a contraceptive method that she can use correctly and consistently.

FACT 3.
A woman who wants to become pregnant again after an abortion or miscarriage should wait 6 months so she can regain strength for her next pregnancy.

Even if her pregnancy was planned and she wants to get pregnant again, after a miscarriage or abortion a woman needs to begin a family planning method

CHAPTER 8: **FAMILY PLANNING AFTER MISCARRIAGE OR ABORTION**

and give her body at least 6 months to regain its strength and prepare for the next pregnancy. Becoming pregnant sooner may lead to health problems for the mother and the baby, such as anemia (low iron level in the blood), another miscarriage, premature birth, or a small or underweight baby.

Starting a contraceptive method immediately after an abortion or miscarriage will help to make sure that the next pregnancy is a healthy one. Couples can choose almost any method. If a woman has an infection, however, IUD insertion or sterilization should be postponed until the infection is cured. She should use another method in the meantime. (For more information on family planning methods, see Chapter 7.)

Health care providers should help women after an abortion or miscarriage to decide on a method that is safe for her. They need to help women avoid a future abortion by helping her understand why the unintended pregnancy occurred, helping her to select a reliable contraceptive method, and encouraging correct and consistent method use.

FACT 4.
To reduce the risk of infection after an abortion or miscarriage, a woman should avoid having sex until all bleeding stops — usually 5 to 7 days. Women who are treated for infection or abortion-related injury need to be sure the vagina or uterus has healed before having sex again.

Light bleeding and spotting is common after an abortion or miscarriage. Couples should wait until this bleeding stops completely and until the woman feels comfortable before having sex again. Typically, the bleeding stops after 5 to 7 days, but it may last up to 2 weeks. If the woman had an injury to her vagina or uterus, or if she is being treated for infection, she should wait until her body is fully healed before having sex.

Unmarried Young People and Unintended Pregnancy

9

INTRODUCTION

Providing contraceptive information and services to unmarried young people is important. Unintended pregnancy can have extreme consequences. Pregnant young women may have to leave school, causing emotional harm and limiting their education. Pregnancy at a young age can also have major physical risks and affect a young woman's status in the family and community.

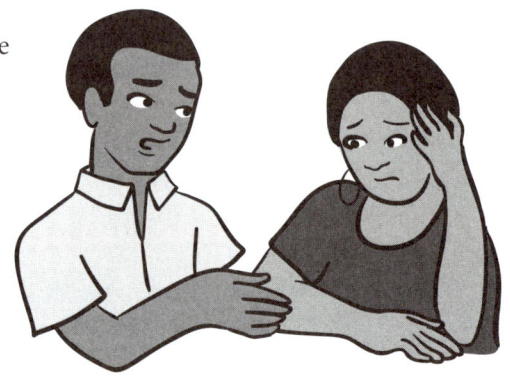

Although most societies discourage sex before marriage, many young people are sexually active before they are married. Often, young people take risks and have a sense that "it can't happen to me." As a result, unmarried girls in their teen years do get pregnant. Many young people do not know about fertility and how to avoid pregnancy and STIs, including HIV.

To avoid unintended pregnancies, young people need appropriate and accurate information about sexuality, fertility, contraception, and STIs/HIV prevention. They also need opportunities to discuss this information and to build important decision-making skills with the help of trained and trusted people. Parents, teachers, community and religious leaders, and trained peer

(Continued on page 82)

KEY FACTS TO SHARE:
UNMARRIED YOUNG PEOPLE AND UNINTENDED PREGNANCY

1 For an unmarried young woman, unintended pregnancy can have extreme consequences. Pregnant young women may have to leave school, causing emotional harm and limiting their education and work opportunities. They may also face serious physical risks.

2 Most young people can use any contraceptive method safely. They need to know the full range of contraceptives available and may need help choosing the method that will suit them best.

3 Complete sexual abstinence is the most effective way to avoid both pregnancy and STIs/HIV. However, abstinence may be hard to practice consistently. Should young people become sexually active, they need to know about contraceptive methods, including condoms and emergency contraception.

4 Young men need to share responsibility for protecting young women from unintended pregnancy and STIs/HIV. They can do so by respecting women's right to say no to sex and not using pressure or violence when they say no. They should use condoms consistently and correctly to prevent STIs/HIV even when their partners are using another contraceptive method to prevent pregnancy.

(Continued on page 83)

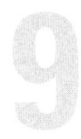

CHAPTER 9: **UNMARRIED YOUNG PEOPLE AND UNINTENDED PREGNANCY**

educators all can be good and trusted sources of information and guidance. These allies of youth need good information themselves.

Sharing information with young people about sexuality, contraception, and other aspects of reproductive health does not increase their sexual activity. In fact, sharing such information and helping young people think about their future helps to delay the start of sexual activity, increases contraceptive use by those already sexually active, lowers the number of sexual partners, and decreases the frequency of sex.

Providers of contraception also have an important role to play — making sexual and reproductive health services easier for young people to obtain. These services need to be welcoming and friendly toward young, single women and men. Being judgmental will not help the young person and can do them harm by scaring them away from getting information and services they need. Providers need to present accurate information and help young people consider their sexual behavior and contraceptive choices. As with all other clients, counseling sessions must be private, and even the fact that the young person has come for services must be kept confidential.

KEY FACTS TO SHARE:
UNMARRIED YOUNG PEOPLE AND UNINTENDED PREGNANCY

5 Young women should be able to identify the days in their menstrual cycle when pregnancy would be most likely. Understanding their fertility helps young women avoid unintended pregnancy and protect their own health. Young men should know that they may cause pregnancy every time they have sex.

6 Young people are at higher risk for STIs/HIV due to their risk-taking behavior. Young women are vulnerable for biological reasons, too. Young people can reduce the risk of STIs/HIV by practicing abstinence, reducing the number of sexual partners, choosing circumcision (for men, to reduce HIV risk), and using condoms correctly and consistently every time they have sex.

CHAPTER 9: UNMARRIED YOUNG PEOPLE AND UNINTENDED PREGNANCY

SUPPORTING INFORMATION

FACT 1.
For an unmarried young woman, unintended pregnancy can have extreme consequences. Pregnant young women may have to leave school, causing emotional harm and limiting their education and work opportunities. They may also face serious physical risks.

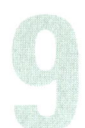

In most cultures young unmarried mothers face stigma that can have harmful psychological and social impact. Pregnancy usually means the end of formal education. Becoming a mother at a young age changes a young woman's life course and often robs her of basic life choices such as jobs, earning capacity, opportunities, and future marriage. Raising a child is a major economic burden. Those who are already poor are more likely to remain in poverty. The consequences of early pregnancy are much more severe for young women than for young men. But some young men also may bear some social and psychological consequences, especially if they leave school to support a child.

Unintended pregnancies among young women often end in unsafe abortion, especially where safe services are not available or affordable. Some young unmarried women risk unsafe abortion rather than face health clinic staff who may judge them. Unsafe abortion often leads to complications that may affect young woman's ability to have children in the future and cause other life-long health problems or even death.

Unintended pregnancy has serious health risks for young women. Those ages 15 through 18 are twice as likely to die during childbirth compared to women ages 20 to 24, and girls under age 15 are 5 times more likely to die

CHAPTER 9: **UNMARRIED YOUNG PEOPLE AND UNINTENDED PREGNANCY**

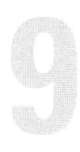

during childbirth. Young women are more likely to have high blood pressure when they are pregnant, which may lead to life-threatening seizures. They may experience a long or blocked labor that often leads to serious bleeding, infection, and other complications, such as fistula.

FACT 2.
Most young people can use any contraceptive method safely. They need to know the full range of contraceptives available and may need help choosing the method that will suit them best.

There are no medical reasons to deny any contraceptive method based on young age alone. Almost all young people can use any method safely. Sterilization is the only method that, while medically safe, is generally not appropriate for young people because it permanently ends fertility. Because young people are at the beginning of their reproductive years, they are likely to want to have children later in life.

Providers should tell young people about all available contraceptive options, without pressure or judgment, and help them make a voluntary decision that is in their own best interest. Together, with young people, providers and counselors need to consider the following factors regarding contraceptive use:

- Unmarried youth may be more likely to engage in risk-taking behavior than older people or even married young people. This behavior includes having multiple sexual partners or changing partners more often. Because of this, most sexually active young people need to think about the risk of STIs/HIV and consider methods that offer protection from both pregnancy and STIs/HIV — that is, approaches that provide "dual protection."

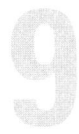

CHAPTER 9: **UNMARRIED YOUNG PEOPLE AND UNINTENDED PREGNANCY**

- One of the most important factors for young people choosing a contraceptive method is how difficult it is to use the method consistently and correctly to ensure effectiveness.

- To be effective, some methods, such as oral contraceptive pills, rely on a woman's ability to use them correctly. Some young women find consistent daily pill-taking difficult. If so, they can choose a method that does not require daily action.

- Implants and IUDs are among the easiest methods to use correctly. Once inserted, they provide highly effective protection for several years. Young women, with or without children, can use these methods safely. Implants are becoming more available in many countries and more popular among young women. IUDs are also a convenient option. An IUD should not be inserted if a young woman has a current infection with gonorrhea or chlamydia or is at very high risk of getting such an infection.

- Injectables can also be an easy method to use, but a young person must remember to get re-injections regularly.

- Some young women may find fertility awareness methods difficult to use if their menstrual cycles are still irregular. Irregular cycles make it hard to accurately identify fertile days. Still, it is valuable for young women to know when they are most likely to be fertile (see Fact 5).

- Condoms are often popular among youth. They provide protection from both pregnancy and STIs/HIV and are easy to obtain. Also, many young people have sex only occasionally, and condoms can be used just when needed. Still, condoms require correct and consistent use, which involves partner cooperation. As a result, condoms are less effective at preventing pregnancy than some other methods. Young women may want to consider using another contraceptive method in addition to condoms to increase protection from pregnancy.

CHAPTER 9: **UNMARRIED YOUNG PEOPLE AND UNINTENDED PREGNANCY**

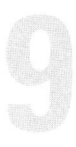

In addition, all young people should be informed about availability of emergency contraception and where to get it. Because sex among youth is often unplanned, they may not be using a regular contraceptive method. Emergency contraception can help to prevent pregnancy after unprotected sex.

FACT 3.
Complete sexual abstinence is the most effective way to avoid both pregnancy and STIs/HIV. However, abstinence may be hard to practice consistently. Should young people become sexually active, they need to know about contraceptive methods, including condoms and emergency contraception.

Complete sexual abstinence provides complete protection from both pregnancy and STIs/HIV. Messages promoting abstinence appear to work best when addressed to young people who are not yet sexually active, especially girls. Some programs that include abstinence messages have delayed the start of sexual activity by about a year.

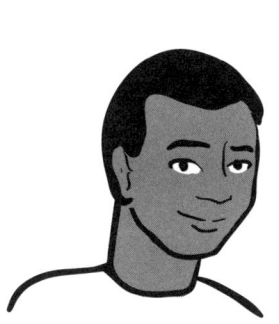
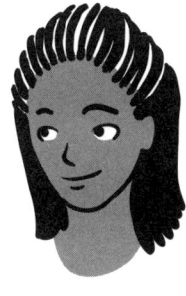

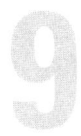

CHAPTER 9: **UNMARRIED YOUNG PEOPLE AND UNINTENDED PREGNANCY**

The term "abstinence" can mean different things to different people. Some view abstinence as a commitment to refrain from sex until marriage. Others view abstinence as delaying sex until some future time — for example, when entering into a committed relationship, possibly before marriage. Or the term can refer to those who have been sexually active at one time but now have decided to abstain from sex for various reasons. Also, some may consider themselves to be practicing abstinence if they avoid vaginal intercourse, even if they engage in other kinds of sexual intimacy. This may avoid pregnancy but not necessarily all STIs/HIV.

In practice, abstaining from sex tends to be less effective in preventing pregnancy than some contraceptive methods because complete abstinence requires strong motivation, self-control, communication, and commitment. A person may have sex in a "weak" moment. Young people need to develop skills to practice abstinence successfully and to say no to unwanted sexual activity.

Because of the challenges of abstinence, young people need to know about other contraceptive options and ways to reduce the risk of STIs/HIV. In many countries comprehensive sexual health programs that encourage abstinence while providing accurate information about contraception and condom use have reduced sexual activity among young people. Such programs also have increased the use of condoms and other contraceptives among sexually active youth.

Young people who practice abstinence require strong social support to be successful. Parents, teachers, trusted community members, and health care providers all have roles to play in motivating youth and helping them to develop communication and negotiation skills. They also need to make sure that young people get accurate information not only about abstinence but also about contraceptive options and about behavior that may risk getting STIs/HIV.

Facts for Family Planning

CHAPTER 9: **UNMARRIED YOUNG PEOPLE AND UNINTENDED PREGNANCY**

FACT 4.
Young men need to share responsibility for protecting young women from unintended pregnancy and STIs/HIV. They can do so by respecting women's right to say no to sex and not using pressure or violence when they say no. They should use condoms consistently and correctly to prevent STIs/HIV even when their partners are using another contraceptive method to prevent pregnancy.

The way that young men and women approach relationships, including sex, often depends on their understanding of society's gender norms — that is, the expectation of how men and women, boys and girls should behave. For girls and women, gender norms in many cultures call for male authority, economic dependence on men, virginity until marriage, and faithfulness during marriage. Norms for men, in contrast, are often built around power and control, independence, not showing emotions, risk-taking, using violence to resolve conflict, early sexual activity, and having multiple sexual partners. Certain gender norms contribute to unintended pregnancy, STIs/HIV, sexual violence and coercion, early marriage, and other harmful behaviors. There are, of course, gender norms that are protective. For instance, the cultural expectation that young women will be virgins at the time of marriage could protect them from pregnancy and getting HIV or other STIs.

Changing harmful norms is difficult but important. All young people, especially young women, have the right to refuse sex and not be coerced or forced into sex. Girls and women are especially at risk for unintended pregnancy and STIs/HIV when sex is forced.

Facts for Family Planning | **89**

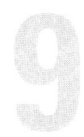

CHAPTER 9: **UNMARRIED YOUNG PEOPLE AND UNINTENDED PREGNANCY**

Real men will share the responsibility for protecting young women from unintended pregnancy and STIs/HIV. They will ask if their partner is using contraception and never simply assume she is protected. Real men are equal partners in preventing pregnancy. They will also take responsibility for avoiding STIs/HIV by using condoms correctly and consistently at each sexual encounter.

Attitudes about gender roles are changing. Messages for young men will continue to encourage these positive changes. Gender norms can guide real men to treat women with respect, share responsibility for sexual and reproductive health decisions, and never be violent to women, including their sister, mother, girlfriend, and wife. Messages for young men should also include not pressuring their male peers to have sex.

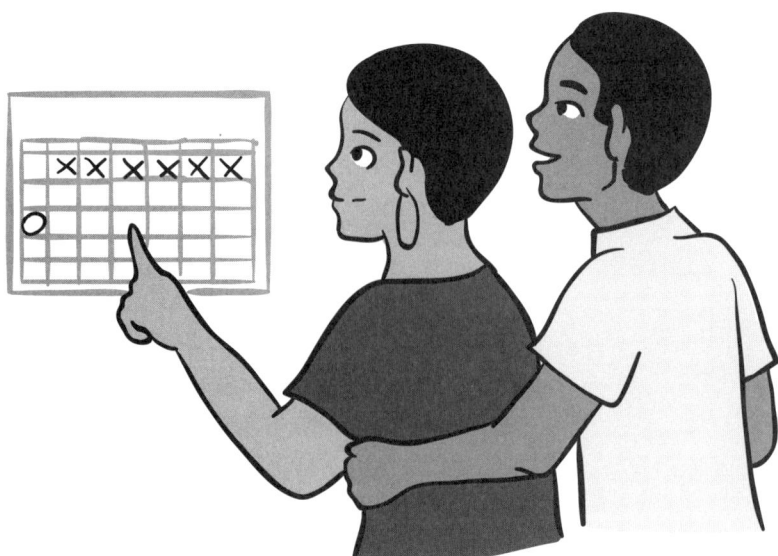

CHAPTER 9: **UNMARRIED YOUNG PEOPLE AND UNINTENDED PREGNANCY**

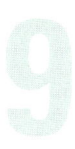

FACT 5.
Young women should be able to identify the days in their menstrual cycle when pregnancy would be most likely. Understanding their fertility helps young women avoid unintended pregnancy and protect their own health. Young men should know that they may cause pregnancy every time they have sex.

All young people need to learn about women's and men's reproductive systems, their fertility, the menstrual cycle, and how pregnancy occurs. They need to understand when they are fertile and thus when sex can lead to pregnancy. For example, boys need to know that they start producing sperm during puberty, which occurs between the ages of 9 and 15. Once this process begins, men's bodies continuously produce sperm. Thus, men are fertile all the time and may cause pregnancy any time they have unprotected sex.

A woman is fertile for several days each month. During these days she can become pregnant if she has unprotected sex. Most women should assume that there is a period of 12 days each month when they could get pregnant. Girls may become fertile for the first time approximately 2 weeks before the first monthly bleeding, which occurs sometime between the ages of 8 and 13 for most girls. Understanding fertility is a way to help young people understand their maturing bodies and know how to protect their own sexual and reproductive health.

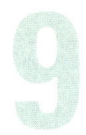

CHAPTER 9: **UNMARRIED YOUNG PEOPLE AND UNINTENDED PREGNANCY**

FACT 6.
Young people are at higher risk for STIs/HIV due to their risk-taking behavior. Young women are vulnerable for biological reasons, too. Young people can reduce the risk of STIs/HIV by practicing abstinence, reducing the number of sexual partners, choosing circumcision (for men, to reduce HIV risk), and using condoms correctly and consistently every time they have sex.

Young people are at high risk of STIs including HIV, and about two of every five new HIV infections occur in young people ages 15 to 24. This is due mostly to risky behavior. Many young men and women are aware of the dangers of HIV, but they often believe that it cannot happen to them. Also, many lack knowledge of other STIs or do not have the communication skills or power to negotiate condom use with a sexual partner. As a result, many young people do not use condoms consistently and correctly. Other high-risk behaviors common among young people include having more than one sexual partner or changing partners often. Also, use of drugs or alcohol can lead to risky behavior.

> Young people can reduce the risk of STIs/HIV by practicing abstinence, reducing the number of sexual partners, choosing circumcision (for men, to reduce HIV risk), and using condoms correctly and consistently every time they have sex.

In addition, there are biological factors that make women in general and young women in particular more likely to get STIs/HIV than men. It is estimated that sexual transmission of HIV from a man to a woman is about twice as likely as transmission from a woman to a man. This is because the female genital tract (vagina) has a much larger surface that may be exposed to HIV during sex than the male genitals (penis). Also, women may be exposed to HIV for a longer period of time than men because semen still remains in the vagina after intercourse ends. Young women may be at higher

CHAPTER 9: **UNMARRIED YOUNG PEOPLE AND UNINTENDED PREGNANCY**

risk of chlamydial infection than older women. This is because a young woman's cervix (the entrance into the uterus) often contains cells that are fragile and especially vulnerable to chlamydial infection.

Young men and women need to know what behaviors increase the risk of STIs/HIV. They also need to know ways to avoid or reduce this risk. These ways include avoiding sex entirely (including oral and anal sex), reducing the number of sexual partners, limiting the number of new partners, staying in a faithful relationship with one uninfected partner, and using condoms correctly with every intercourse. Young men should also consider getting circumcised because circumcision reduces a man's risk of getting HIV during vaginal sex with a woman. However, young men should know that even when circumcised they must continue using condoms because the possibility of HIV transmission still remains.

Family Planning and Sexually Transmitted Infections, including HIV

INTRODUCTION

To protect themselves, people need correct information about sexually transmitted infections (STIs), including HIV. Women and men of all ages should know what situations and behaviors increase their chances of exposure to STIs/HIV. They also need to know how to protect themselves and others from these infections. Ways to avoid STIs/HIV are:

- Never have sex (abstain)
- Have sex only with one uninfected partner who also has no other sexual partners
- Always use condoms and use them correctly

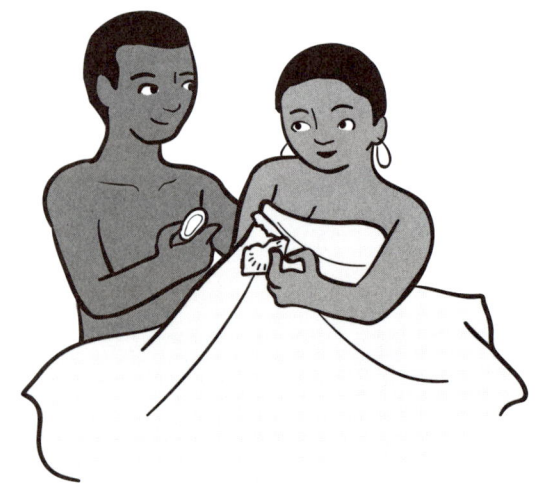

Ways to lower risk, but not entirely avoid risk, are:

- Have fewer sexual partners
- For young people, delay the start of sexual activity
- Boys and men can choose to get circumcised

(Continued on page 96)

94 | Facts for Family Planning

KEY FACTS TO SHARE:
FAMILY PLANNING AND SEXUALLY TRANSMITTED INFECTIONS, INCLUDING HIV

1. People can avoid getting or transmitting STIs/HIV if they do not have sex; if they have sex only with one faithful, uninfected partner; or if they consistently and correctly use condoms during every sex act.

2. By having fewer sexual partners, people can lower their chances of getting STIs/HIV, but not completely avoid all risk. Young people also can lower their chances of infection by delaying the start of sexual activity. In addition, uncircumcised men can get circumcised to greatly lower their chances of getting HIV during vaginal sex with an HIV infected woman.

3. When men and women get tested for HIV, they can discuss the results with their sexual partners and decide together on the kind of protection they need.

4. People who need protection from both pregnancy and STIs/HIV can consider using two methods together: condoms for STIs/HIV protection and a highly effective contraceptive method for added protection from pregnancy. People can also choose to rely on using condoms consistently and correctly to prevent both pregnancy and infection.

(Continued on page 97)

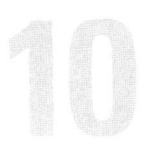

CHAPTER 3: **FAMILY PLANNING AND SEXUALLY TRANSMITTED INFECTIONS, INCLUDING HIV**

Sexually active couples often want to avoid pregnancy and also want to protect themselves from STIs/HIV. They need to know how to meet both needs — called "dual protection." Some couples use condoms alone to prevent both pregnancy and infection. Other couples use condoms for protection from STIs/HIV and also use a highly effective family planning method for added protection from pregnancy.

People who already have an STI, including HIV, can use almost any contraceptive method safely. There are only a few health issues related to STIs/HIV that may affect a woman's contraceptive choice. People with STIs/HIV should also use condoms correctly every time they have sex to avoid infecting sexual partners.

> Preventing unintended pregnancies among women living with HIV is the most cost-effective way of preventing HIV transmission from mother to child.

In some couples, one or both partners are living with HIV, and they want to have a baby. A knowledgeable health care provider can help these couples to lower the risk of passing HIV to their baby or to an uninfected partner and understand how to have a healthy pregnancy.

KEY FACTS TO SHARE:
FAMILY PLANNING AND SEXUALLY TRANSMITTED INFECTIONS, INCLUDING HIV

5 Almost all contraceptive methods are safe for people with STIs, including HIV. However, some hormonal methods may be less effective when a woman takes certain drugs for treatment of HIV or tuberculosis. Other methods should not be started until a woman's health improves. A health care provider will help a woman to make the best choice.

6 If one or both partners in a couple are living with HIV and they want to have a baby, the safest time for unprotected sex is when the partner with HIV is in good health and receives antiretroviral therapy (if available). Also, the couple should have sex without a condom only during the woman's fertile days.

7 Pregnant women with HIV can lower the chances of passing HIV to their babies by taking antiretroviral drugs (ARVs) and giving ARVs to the baby immediately after birth. These women should also have regular health care before the baby is born and give birth with the help of a skilled health care provider to increase their chances of having a healthy baby.

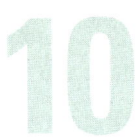

CHAPTER 3: **FAMILY PLANNING AND SEXUALLY TRANSMITTED INFECTIONS, INCLUDING HIV**

SUPPORTING INFORMATION

FACT 1.
People can avoid getting or transmitting STIs/HIV if they do not have sex; if they have sex only with one faithful, uninfected partner; or if they consistently and correctly use condoms during every sex act.

Not everyone faces exposure to STIs/HIV. In fact, many people who need or use family planning are in stable relationships and have no other sex partners, or they live in areas where few others are infected with HIV. They face little or no risk of HIV or other STIs. Still, everyone should know what behavior to avoid in order to decrease their risk. Behaviors that can increase exposure to STIs/HIV include:

- Sex with more than one partner

- Sex with a partner who has other sexual partners and does not correctly and consistently use condoms

- Sex with a partner who has STI symptoms (for example, discharge from penis, unusual vaginal discharge, burning or pain during urination, lower abdominal pain or pain during sex, swollen or painful testicles, sores on the genitals)

- Having a partner who has recently been diagnosed or treated for an STI/HIV

- Not using condoms correctly and consistently with a new partner (especially when living in a community where STIs are common).

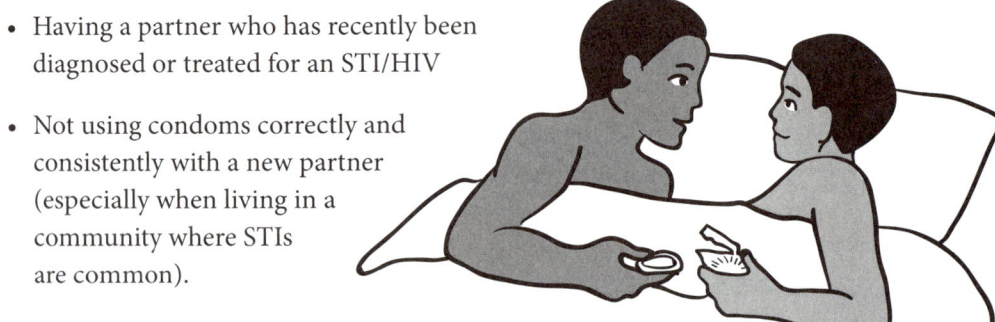

CHAPTER 3: **FAMILY PLANNING AND SEXUALLY TRANSMITTED INFECTIONS, INCLUDING HIV**

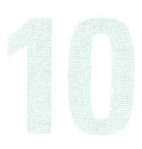

One sure way to avoid getting an infection through sex is to abstain completely from sex. For many people, however, this may not be a realistic choice. For those who do have sex, sex with only one partner — who is also uninfected — will avoid STIs/HIV infection. In this case both partners must be tested and found to have no infection, must tell each other their test results, and must remain faithful to each other. When partners do not know their own or each other's infection status, or when one or both partners are infected, correct and consistent condom use is a reliable way to prevent the transmission of infection between partners.

To decide together how to prevent infection, couples need to discuss openly their sexual relationship, risky behaviors, infection status, and the possibility of getting tested. They should also be able to discuss and make joint decisions about condom use.

FACT 2.
By having fewer sexual partners, people can lower their chances of getting STIs/HIV, but not completely avoid all risk. Young people also can lower their chances of infection by delaying the start of sexual activity. In addition, uncircumcised men can get circumcised to greatly lower their chances of getting HIV during vaginal sex with an HIV infected woman.

Reducing the number of sexual partners has been part of all successful strategies to limit the spread of HIV. Having fewer partners does not avoid all risk of exposure to STIs/HIV, but it does lower the chances of being infected. In general, people should consider reducing their number of sexual partners along with taking other preventive steps. Having only one sexual partner, who is uninfected, is best.

Facts for Family Planning

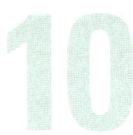

CHAPTER 3: **FAMILY PLANNING AND SEXUALLY TRANSMITTED INFECTIONS, INCLUDING HIV**

Young people reduce their chances of STIs/HIV infection when they postpone the start of sexual activity. As they get older, they will develop stronger personal and social skills to recognize and avoid risky situations and to negotiate for protection during sex. Also, young people who have already started having sex can decide to stop for a time and so avoid the risk. Whether or not they have ever had sex, all young people need accurate information so that they know how to avoid STIs/HIV infection when they start having sex.

Circumcision lowers a man's risk of getting HIV during vaginal sex. Male circumcision is a simple surgical procedure. It involves removing the foreskin, the loose fold of skin that covers the head of the penis. The foreskin creates a moist environment where HIV can survive longer. Also, the foreskin contains cells that are especially vulnerable to infection by HIV. Circumcision can be done at any stage of life — during infancy, childhood, adolescence, or adulthood.

Circumcision lowers a man's risk of getting HIV infection from a woman by at least 60%. Circumcised men still can get HIV infection, however. A man who chooses to be circumcised for HIV protection should continue using other protection strategies, too, such as correct and consistent condom use and reducing the number of sexual partners.

FACT 3.
When men and women get tested for HIV, they can discuss the results with their sexual partners and decide together on the kind of protection they need.

People can benefit from knowing their HIV status. Knowing their HIV status will help them to make informed decisions about sexual behavior, condom use, other contraceptive methods, having children, and other health issues

CHAPTER 3: **FAMILY PLANNING AND SEXUALLY TRANSMITTED INFECTIONS, INCLUDING HIV**

such as nutrition, medication, rest, and exercise. Whether the test results are positive or negative, knowing them will help people live healthier lives. To learn their status, people need to know where to get HIV testing and counseling and to be able to use these services without stigma and discrimination.

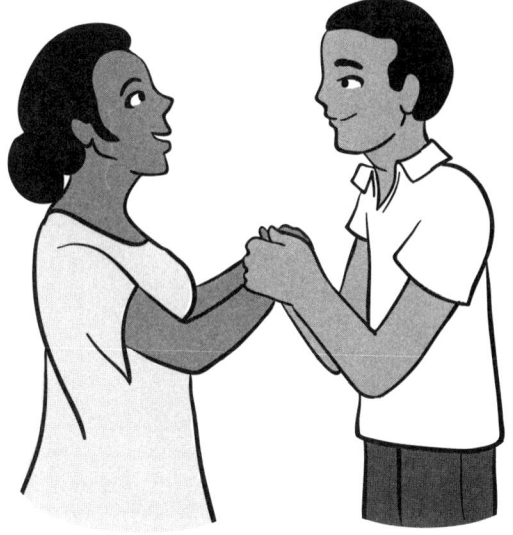

Counselors specifically trained to counsel couples can help couples discuss these often-sensitive issues. Counselors and health care providers also can help individuals and couples understand approaches to safer sex, help them practice condom negotiation, and either provide or know where to refer them for testing or treatment for STIs/HIV. A person who suspects that his or her partner may have HIV should get tested and use condoms correctly and consistently during sex. A request to use condoms does not mean that one does not trust one's partner. Because a person can get HIV several years before symptoms appear, the couple may be in a faithful relationship now, while one partner may have been infected long before they met.

Persons living with HIV can still live long and happy lives. They should discuss with their counselors and health care providers the possibility of starting antiretroviral therapy. Antiretroviral therapy is a lifelong medication course that helps to control HIV infection, although it does not eliminate it. People with HIV should also continue using condoms correctly and consistently even if their partners are also infected. Condoms will help protect

Facts for Family Planning

CHAPTER 3: **FAMILY PLANNING AND SEXUALLY TRANSMITTED INFECTIONS, INCLUDING HIV**

them from another type of HIV or another STI that can make them sicker. They should also use condoms to protect partners who may not have HIV.

FACT 4.
People who need protection from both pregnancy and STIs/HIV can consider using two methods together: condoms for STIs/HIV protection and a highly effective contraceptive method for added protection from pregnancy. People can also choose to rely on using condoms consistently and correctly to prevent both pregnancy and infection.

Many couples' choice of contraception should take into account both preventing pregnancy and preventing STIs/HIV. Male and female condoms are the only contraceptive methods that provide STIs/HIV protection. However, condoms are less effective for preventing pregnancy than many other contraceptive methods — about 85% effective as typically used.

A couple may choose to use both condoms and a more effective contraceptive method in order to achieve dual protection. Some couples use two methods successfully, but others may feel less motivated to use two methods or may have difficulties using one or both methods consistently and correctly. Also, using two methods may be more expensive or harder to acquire.

Other couples may choose to rely on condoms alone to protect against STIs/HIV and pregnancy. This requires using a male or female condom correctly with every act of sex. When used correctly and consistently, male condoms are 98% effective protecting against pregnancy; female condoms are 95% effective. Similarly, when condoms are used consistently and correctly for every sex act, they prevent 80% to 95% of HIV infections that would have occurred without condom use. Condoms are an inexpensive contraceptive

CHAPTER 3: **FAMILY PLANNING AND SEXUALLY TRANSMITTED INFECTIONS, INCLUDING HIV**

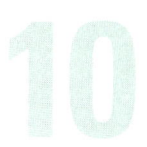

and easy to find. Couples who are highly motivated to use them correctly and consistently every time they have sex can prevent pregnancy and protect themselves against STIs.

Providers can help clients decide which approach to preventing pregnancy and STIs/HIV will best suit them.

FACT 5.
Almost all contraceptive methods are safe for people with STIs, including HIV. However, some hormonal methods may be less effective when a woman takes certain drugs for treatment of HIV or tuberculosis. Other methods should not be started until a woman's health improves. A health care provider will help a woman to make the best choice.

People with STIs and people living with HIV can use most contraceptive methods safely and effectively. One exception is spermicides, including a diaphragm with spermicides. A women at risk of HIV and women with HIV/AIDS who frequently have sex should not use spermicides because frequent use of spermicides can increase the chances of getting HIV or being infected with another type of HIV.

There are also a few issues to consider when selecting a contraceptive method:

- Oral contraceptive pills and combined injectable contraceptives, often called monthly injectables, may be less effective for women who take certain antiretroviral drugs for HIV, or some drugs for tuberculosis, which often accompanies HIV infection.

- An IUD should not be inserted if a woman has gonorrhea or chlamydial infection, or if her health is poor because of AIDS.

Facts for Family Planning | 103

CHAPTER 3: **FAMILY PLANNING AND SEXUALLY TRANSMITTED INFECTIONS, INCLUDING HIV**

- Female and male sterilization should be delayed if an individual has an active STI or AIDS-related illness until the condition is cured or health improves.

Health care providers will help people decide if and when they can start safely and effectively using the contraceptive method of their choice. In addition, people who might get HIV or another STI or who are infected should always be advised that male and female condoms are the only contraceptive methods that prevent the transmission of STIs/HIV.

FACT 6.
If one or both partners in a couple are living with HIV and they want to have a baby, the safest time for unprotected sex is when the partner with HIV is in good health and receives antiretroviral therapy (if available). Also, the couple should have sex without a condom only during the woman's fertile days.

Health care providers can help couples with HIV to decide when the right time for pregnancy is and to learn how to reduce the chances of transmitting HIV while trying to get pregnant. When one partner, but not the other, has HIV and the couple is planning to have a baby, it is important to try to get pregnant when the partner living with HIV is in good health. Good health means that the body's defense system is stronger and can fight HIV better. This lowers the chances that HIV will be transmitted between partners and to the baby. If health is good, and there are no signs or symptoms of HIV disease or infections (for example, tuberculosis), the chances for a healthy pregnancy and a healthy baby are good. If, instead, the health of the partner with HIV is getting worse or is poor, unprotected sex should be delayed until treatment can be given and health improves. An HIV-infected partner (man or woman) should start antiretroviral therapy prior to trying to achieve

CHAPTER 3: **FAMILY PLANNING AND SEXUALLY TRANSMITTED INFECTIONS, INCLUDING HIV**

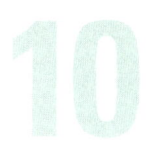

pregnancy. This will minimize the risk of HIV transmission to the uninfected partner and to the child.

When one partner is infected and the other is not, the safest way for the woman to conceive is for the couple to stop using condoms only during a woman's fertile time of the month and to use condoms at all other times. Sex without condom use outside fertile days will increase the risk of HIV infection, but it will not increase the chances of pregnancy.

Health care providers can help couples with HIV decide when is the right time to try to become pregnant and how to minimize the risk of HIV transmission.

FACT 7.
Pregnant women with HIV can lower the chances of passing HIV to their babies by taking antiretroviral drugs (ARVs) and giving ARVs to the baby immediately after birth. These women should also have regular health care before the baby is born and give birth with the help of a skilled health care provider to increase their chances of having a healthy baby.

HIV can be transmitted from mother to child during pregnancy, labor, delivery, or breastfeeding. Without medical help, 25% to 40% of infants born to mothers with HIV will become infected. With proper care by a health care provider, this risk can be reduced to less than 5%. Thus, HIV transmission from a pregnant woman to her infant can often be prevented.

A woman with HIV lowers the chances that her baby will get HIV when she stays as healthy as possible. At regular health care visits before the baby is born, this woman will receive all the basic pregnancy care given to uninfected women as well as special care to help her maintain her overall health.

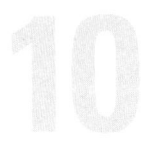

CHAPTER 3: **FAMILY PLANNING AND SEXUALLY TRANSMITTED INFECTIONS, INCLUDING HIV**

Also, a pregnant woman with HIV can get ARV medicines that greatly reduce the chances that her baby will be born with HIV. The health care providers will decide when to start this treatment and what drugs to use. A short course of antiretroviral therapy — 4 to 6 weeks — should also be given to infants born to HIV-infected mothers to minimize the risk of HIV transmission.

Finally, women with HIV need to give birth at a health center. For their part, health workers at the facilities need to take special care to prevent HIV from being passed from the mother to babies during birth. They also can help mothers decide how best to feed the baby and give advice on nutrition. While baby formula eliminates the possibility of passing HIV to the baby in breast milk, baby formula may not be a realistic or safe choice in countries without reliable and affordable access to baby formula or without clean drinking water. Where reliable, affordable, and safe formula-feeding is not an option, the best choice for the baby is exclusive breastfeeding for the first 6 months.

Women with HIV who are pregnant or considering pregnancy should know where to get health care services before the baby is born and should be encouraged to do so as soon as possible. At the same time, men should be encouraged to learn how to support their partners throughout pregnancy, as well as during and after delivery. Male partners can influence women to be tested for HIV and to use health care services before the baby is born. In fact, when woman have their partners' support, rates of HIV transmission from mother to child are lower.

Glossary of Terms

ANEMIA: Anemia has many causes, but two common ones are bleeding and poor nutrition. This condition reduces the capacity of the blood to carry oxygen, because a person has a lower-than-normal number of red blood cells or low hemoglobin (a chemical substance responsible for transporting oxygen in the blood). People with anemia may feel tired, fatigue easily, appear pale, develop rapid or pounding heart beats, and become short of breath.

ANTIRETROVIRAL DRUGS: Also referred to as ARVs, these are medications for the treatment of infections by a certain types of viruses called "retroviruses." One of the most common retroviruses is HIV. ARVs help to manage and control HIV by slowing down its ability to multiply.

ANTIRETROVIRAL THERAPY: Standard antiretroviral therapy (ART) consists of the combination of at least three antiretroviral drugs (ARVs). The combination of ARVs makes it harder for HIV to multiply. Antiretroviral therapy cannot cure HIV, but it can stop the progression of HIV disease. It can also prevent transmission of HIV from mother to child when taken by a mother during pregnancy and given to the baby after delivery.

CERVIX: The cervix is the narrow part of the uterus, which opens into the vagina. The cervix has strong, thick walls. The opening of the cervix is very small (smaller than a straw). During childbirth, the cervix expands to allow a baby to pass.

CIRCUMCISION: This simple surgical procedure involves removing the foreskin — the loose fold of skin that covers the head of the penis. The foreskin contains cells that are especially vulnerable to infection by HIV. The foreskin also creates a moist environment where HIV can survive longer. Removing the foreskin reduces a man's risk of getting HIV infection during vaginal sex with a woman by at least 60%.

CONTRACEPTION: The intentional prevention of pregnancy through the use of various drugs, devices, surgical procedures, or sexual practices.

CONTRACEPTIVE METHODS: Various drugs, devices, surgical procedures, or sexual practices used to prevent pregnancy.

GLOSSARY OF TERMS

DEATH RATE: The number of deaths per 1,000 of the population per year.

EGG (OR OVUM): The reproductive cell of the female.

EJACULATION: The release of semen from the opening at the tip of the penis when a man reaches sexual climax (orgasm).

FAITHFUL PARTNER OR FAITHFUL RELATIONSHIPS: These terms refer to having sexual relations only with your partner, and your partner has no other sexual partners but you.

FALLOPIAN TUBES: These are two narrow tubes that are attached to the upper part of the uterus. They serve as tunnels for the egg to travel from the ovaries to the uterus. Fallopian tubes are the place where the egg unites with a sperm.

FERTILITY: The ability to get pregnant or cause pregnancy.

FERTILIZATION: The process during which a sperm unites with an egg. Fertilization takes place in the fallopian tube.

FISTULA: A severe medical condition in which a hole called a fistula develops between the vagina and either the rectum or the bladder. A fistula can develop during childbirth, usually when a woman is in labor for 12 hours or longer and no skilled provider is available to assist her.

INFERTILITY: Inability to get pregnant or cause pregnancy. A couple is considered to be infertile if pregnancy has not occurred after 12 months of regular sexual activity without the use of contraception (including the delay of return to fertility after stopping use of injectable contraceptives).

LONG-ACTING CONTRACEPTIVE METHODS: Methods that provide effective contraception for an extended period of time (at least a year) without requiring user action. They are the most effective reversible methods of contraception and include IUDs and implants.

MENOPAUSE: The time in woman's life when monthly bleedings permanently stop and a woman no longer ovulates. Menopause is confirmed when there has been no menstrual bleedings for 12 consecutive months and no other cause can be identified. It typically occurs sometime between the ages of 45 and 55 and marks the end of fertility.

GLOSSARY OF TERMS

MENSTRUAL CYCLE: The recurring series of changes in a woman's body that occur every month. During each cycle an egg is produced and the lining of the uterus prepares for pregnancy; if pregnancy does not occur the lining is shed in form of monthly bleeding. Typical menstrual cycles are between 26 and 32 days.

OVARIES: Two small organs, which are located inside a woman's abdomen, one ovary on each side of the uterus. The ovaries grow, store, and release eggs into the fallopian tubes; typically one egg is released by one of the ovaries every month. The ovaries also produce female sex hormones.

OVULATION: The release of the ripe egg from the ovary. Ovulation occurs about two weeks before woman's monthly bleeding.

PENIS: The male reproductive organ used in sexual intercourse. The head of the penis has a small opening, which connects to the urethra — the tube that transports semen and urine. When a man is sexually aroused, the penis becomes erect (stiff). At this point the flow of urine is blocked from the urethra, allowing only semen to be expelled when the man reaches sexual climax (orgasm).

PERMANENT CONTRACEPTIVE METHODS: These methods include female and male sterilization and are intended to end a woman's or a man's ability to have children permanently.

PUBERTY: The stage of adolescence in which bodies gradually change and become capable of getting pregnant (girls) or causing pregnancy (boys).

REVERSIBLE CONTRACEPTIVE METHODS: These methods do not permanently affect a woman's ability to have children. When a couple decides to stop using the method, the woman may become pregnant soon. All contraceptive methods other than male and female sterilization are reversible.

SCROTUM: The loose pouch-like sac of skin that hangs behind and below the penis. It contains the testicles (also called testes).

SEMEN: The thick white fluid that contains sperm and is expelled when the man reaches sexual climax (orgasm).

SEXUAL INTERCOURSE: This term usually refers to the insertion of a man's penis into a woman's vagina. This term may also be used to describe other sexual penetrative acts, such as anal sex or oral sex, which may occur between a man and a woman, two men, or two women.

GLOSSARY OF TERMS

SEXUALLY TRANSMITTED INFECTIONS (STIs): These are infections generally acquired by sexual contact. The organisms that cause STIs may pass from person to person in semen or vaginal fluids, or through genital contact. Some of these infections can also be transmitted non-sexually, such as from mother to infant during pregnancy or childbirth, or through blood transfusions or shared needles.

SHORT-ACTING CONTRACEPTIVE METHODS: Methods that provide effective contraception for a short period of time. Depending on the method, they require user action either every time a couple has sex, every day, every month, or every 2 or 3 months. The examples of such methods include condoms, oral contraceptive pills, and injectables.

SPERM: The reproductive cell of the male.

STILLBORN: Refers to a baby who is born dead after 24 completed weeks of pregnancy.

TESTICLES: Two small oval organs that lie in the scrotum. The testicles produce and store sperm. They also produce testosterone, the primary male sex hormone.

UNPROTECTED SEX: Sexual intercourse when no contraception is used to prevent a pregnancy or no condom is used to prevent STIs, including HIV. Unprotected sex may refer to vaginal sex, anal sex, or oral sex.

UTERUS: The uterus is a hollow, pear-shaped organ that is located inside a woman's abdomen. The uterus holds a developing baby during pregnancy and has a lining, which helps to nourish a baby. When a woman is not pregnant, this lining is shed every month in the form of monthly bleeding. The muscular walls of the uterus are able to expand and contract to accommodate a growing baby and then help push the baby out during labor. When a woman is not pregnant, the uterus is only about 3 inches (7.5 centimeters) long and 2 inches (5 centimeters) wide.

VAGINA: The vagina is a canal that joins the cervix (the lower part of uterus) to the outside of the body. It also is known as the birth canal. The vagina is about 3 to 5 inches (8 to 12 centimeters) long in a grown woman. Because it has muscular walls, it can expand and contract. This ability to expand allows a baby to pass through the vagina during delivery.

VAS DEFERENS: The vas deferens is a long, muscular tube that transports mature sperm from each testicle to the urethra (which is a tube that carries sperm and urine to the tip of the penis).

Selected Resources

A Guide to Family Planning for Community Health Workers and their Clients.
Geneva: World Health Organization (WHO), 2012. Available at: **http://www.who.int/ reproductivehealth/publications/family_planning/9789241503754/en/index.html**

A Summary Report of New Evidence that Gender Perspectives Improve Reproductive Health Outcomes. U.S. Agency for International Development (USAID) and Interagency Gender Working Group. Washington, DC: Population Reference Bureau, 2011. Available at: **http://www.prb.org/igwg_media/summary-report-gender-perspectives.pdf**

Facts for Life. Third edition. UNICEF, WHO, UNESCO, UNFPA, UNDP, UNAIDS, WFP, and the World Bank. New York: UNICEF, 2010. Available at: **http://www.who.int/ nutrition/publications/infantfeeding/factsoflife/en/index.html**

Family Planning: A Global Handbook for Providers. WHO Department of Reproductive Health and Research (WHO/RHR), Johns Hopkins Bloomberg School of Public Health/Center for Communication Programs (CCP), and USAID. Baltimore and Geneva: JHU/CCP and WHO, 2011. Available at: **http://whqlibdoc.who.int/ publications/2011/9780978856373_eng.pdf**

Family Planning and the Environment: Stabilizing Population Would Help Sustain the Planet. UNFPA Fact Sheet, no date. Available at: **http://www.unfpa.org/rh/planning/ mediakit/docs/sheet3.pdf**

Family Planning Saves Lives. Fourth Edition. Rhonda Smith, Lori Ashford, Jay Gribble, and Donna Clifton. Washington, DC: Population Reference Bureau, 2009. Available at: **http://www.prb.org/Reports/2009/fpsl.aspx**

Family Planning: the Unfinished Agenda. John Cleland, Stan Bernstein, et al. The Lancet Sexual and Reproductive Health Series, October 2006. Available at: **http://cdrwww.who.int/ reproductivehealth/publications/general/lancet_3.pdf**

Healthy Timing and Spacing Pregnancies: A Pocket Guide for Health Practitioners, Program Manager, and Community Leaders. Extending Service Delivery Project, no date. Available at: **http://www.esdproj.org/site/DocServer/ESD_PG_spreads.pdf?docID=141**

Powerful Partners: Adolescent Girls' Education and Delayed Childbearing. Elaine Murphy and Dara Carr. Washington, DC: Population Reference Bureau, 2007. Available at: **http://www.prb.org/pdf07/powerfulpartners.pdf**

SELECTED RESOURCES

Report of a WHO Technical Consultation on Birth Spacing. Geneva: WHO, 2007. Available at: **http://www.who.int/reproductivehealth/publications/family_planning/ WHO_RHR_07_1/en/index.html**)

Repositioning Family Planning: Guidelines for Advocacy Action. WHO, Regional Office for Africa, and USAID. 2008. Available at: **http://www.who.int/reproductivehealth/ publications/family_planning/fp_advocacy_tool/en/index.html**